CICATRICIAL PEMPHIGOID

CICATRICIAL PEMPHIGOID

C. Stephen Foster, MD, FACS

CICATRICIAL PEMPHIGOID

C. Stephen Foster MD

Additional editing services performed by Jordan Ueberroth MD

ISBN-13: 978-0-9994905-6-3

(also available in eBook format)

OIUF

THE OCULAR IMMUNOLOGY
AND UVEITIS FOUNDATION

Dedicated to Eye Disease Cure and Education

Acknowledgements /Foreword

I gratefully acknowledge the superb technical assistance of Carolyn De Siena, Beverly Rice, and Julie Daigle, and the dedicated secretarial assistance of Janet Hunter. I am indebted to Dr Peter Wells for his collaborative support and for his editorial assistance in preparation of this manuscript.

INTRODUCTION

Cicatricial Pemphigoid (CP) is a distinct disease entity of unknown but presumed autoimmune cause. Its effect on the eyes is characterized by chronic cicatrizing conjunctivitis, progressive conjunctival subepithelial fibrosis, and resultant fornix foreshortening, symblepharon formation, trichiasis, distichiasis, meibomian duct obstruction, and eventual lacrimal duct compromise with reduced tear supply to the ocular surface. It is of substantial ophthalmologic interest because of its bilaterality, and because it eventually results in legal blindness due to corneal scarring in a high proportion of people with the disease. No topical therapy is effective in stopping the progression of scarring of the conjunctiva. High doses of systemic prednisone can control the process, but the long-term consequences of moderate-to-high doses of systemic steroid required for control of CP are unacceptable. Systemic immunosuppressive therapy, alone or in combination with systemic dapsone, is highly effective in controlling the disease, and may cure it in many instances.

These clinical characteristics coupled with the ocular and the systemic immunopathologic correlates in patients with CP show it to be a systemic disease, and most evidence strongly suggests it is caused or propagated by a defect in immunoregulation.

CP has been one of the main interests of our research group for the past decade. Struck by the catastrophic consequences of this disease, the total lack of efficacy of conventional therapy, and the circumstantial evidence suggesting that CP is an autoimmune disorder, we made a major commitment to the care and study of patients with CP.

The studies have been both clinical and basic, and the care has involved personal responsibility not only for the ocular therapy but also for the systemic management and monitoring of the patients.

The purpose of this thesis is to describe the results of our experience with 130 patients with CP. We have previously published two reports on uncontrolled clinical trials of immunosuppressive therapy for progressive CP affecting the eyes[1,2]; data from those studies are not included here. Many of the results of our studies have been presented publically at scientific meetings, but have been withheld from publication pending submission of this thesis.

Briefly, the findings reported herein are summarized: CP is a systemic autoimmune disorder which produces conjunctival inflammation, progressive subepithelial fibrosis, and eventual visual loss secondary to keratopathy. Its progression can be halted only through systemic chemotherapeutic strategies. It is not a dry-eye syndrome or a mucin-deficient disorder primarily; tear deficiency and mucin deficiency occur late in the course of CP, and these features are secondary consequences to the primary inflammatory and cicatrizing process. Our histopathologic and immunopathologic studies suggest the possibility of a defect in immunoregulation, perhaps with inadequate suppressor T-cell participation, with resultant autoantibody production and chronic inflammatory processes within the substantia propria of the conjunctiva. Inflammatory mediators within the conjunctiva and in the preocular tear film, we believe, produce the morphologic and physiologic changes seen in this tissue, including fibroblast activation, proliferation, and collagen synthesis with cicatrix formation. Reconstructive adnexal/lid surgery and cataract surgery can be safely performed on CP patients after successful control of all inflammatory activity through systemic chemotherapy.

HISTORICAL SURVEY

CLINICAL

Although a Boston dermatologist, Lever,[3] was the first to make the clinical and histopathologic distinction between pemphigoid and pemphigus in his now classic 1953 monograph, CP has undoubtedly existed since ancient times. Lever and Talbott[4] credit Hippocrates[5] with the first use of the word pemphigoid. (Hippocrates described different types of fevers, including a pemphigoid fever, pemphigodes pyretoi, which was probably a fever accompanied by blisters; the original connotation of the root word pemphix was air, puff, breath, or perhaps swelling or blister.) Lever believes, however, that the bullous eruptions described in Hippocrates' writings were not pemphigus or pemphigoid and that these diseases were unknown to him. Lever credits the 18th century physician, Koenig[6] of Berne, Switzerland, with the first written description of pemphigus and Wichmann[7] with the first description of pemphigoid affecting the conjunctiva. Wichmann,[7] as well as Cooper,[8] in 1857, considered the disease affecting the eyes to be pemphigus. Thost[9] and others continued to use the word pemphigus, first coined by deSauvages[10] in 1768. Duke-Elder[11] credits Cooper[8] with the first *adequate* description of CP affecting the eyes; Cooper named the disorder pemphigus of the conjunctiva. von Graefe[12] first described the clinical course and devastating end stage ocular consequences of CP. In 1878 von Kries[13] named the disease essential contraction of the conjunctiva, and the name debate, which continued for approximately a century, began. Ocular pemphigus,[14] essential shrinkage of the conjunctiva,[15] cicatricial ocular pemphigus,[16] benign mucus membrane pemphigoid,[17] chronic pemphigus of the mucus membranes,[18] chronic cicatricial conjunctivitis,[19] and mucosynechiant conjunctivitis[20] are some of the names used to describe this disease. The work of Lever[3] and others clearly demonstrates that the disease examined in this thesis is a form of pemphigoid; CP is the preferred name. Ocular CP, a name commonly used today, is slightly misleading, since the disease is unquestionably systemic, and, as will be seen later, frequently has extraocular manifestations.

In 1900, Franke[15] published a report summarizing the largest series to date of cases of CP affecting the eyes (107); 102 of these 107 cases were previously published case reports, and 5 of them were cases personally followed and treated by Franke. All authors agree that the disease is invariably progressive and that the ultimate prognosis is quite poor. It may take the disease 10 to 30 years or more to reach end stage, with bilateral blindness the result; but if one follows patients with CP on conventional therapy long enough, one will invariably observe the long-term devastating consequences.[11] The progression of the disease, though usually slow, may be punctuated by periods of remission or by periods of explosive exacerbation with rapid progression of conjunctival scarring and associated keratopathy.[11,21] It is also clear that the more advanced the disease is, the more likely it is to progress significantly within 2 years.[22]

CP is probably not quite as rare as published incidence figures indicate. Bittelheim et al[23] estimated 1 in 15,000 ophthalmic patients; Hardy and Lamb[24] and others[11,15] estimated an incidence of 1 in 20,000 patients. Smith and colleagues[25] estimated 1 in 46,000. Bedell[26] estimated 1 in 8000, and Lever and Talbott[4] stated frankly that it is impossible to make an accurate estimate from available data; they guess that the incidence of CP is somewhere between 1 in 12,000 and 1 in 60,000 ophthalmic patients. But these figures estimate the incidence of relatively advanced CP. Diagnosis of this disorder in its early stages is difficult,[11] and most cases are not recognized as CP until they reach what we would categorize as stage III disease. There are, therefore, patients with stage I and stage II CP uncounted in the epidemiologic estimates.

Data on the average age of CP patients are also somewhat distorted by subtleties of the diagnostic signs. CP is said in many publications to be a disease of older people, with average age given as 60[19] or 70 years.[11] Although reports of CP in children may in fact represent cases of localized erythema multiformi, we certainly now recognize that CP can begin at least as early as the third decade of life.

Most reports describe a slight but clear female predilection. Thus, Klauder and Cowan[14] reported 8 females and 3 males, Lever[3] reported

3 females for every male, and Hardy et al[27] reported 52 females and 29 males with CP; 62 of these patients had ocular involvement, but Hardy et al[27] did not report the sex distribution for this subset of patients. No racial or geographic predilection is reported.[27]

OCULAR MANIFESTATIONS

Ocular involvement with CP usually begins as a unilateral conjunctivitis which persists into a chronic condition. Symptoms during this time are typically those of ocular irritation with sensations of ocular burning, and excess tearing and mucus production. Reported signs include conjunctival suffusion, with vascular dilatation, tearing, excess mucus thread in the inferior fornix, and patches of ocular surface epitheliopathy (especially of the conjunctiva), demonstrated best by patchy uptake of 1% rose bengal dye. Additional, more subtle signs, described in detail later, include subepithelial fibrosis with fine, white perivascular stria formation[11] (most easily observed under the inferior and the superior tarsal conjunctival epithelium) and conjunctival thickening with cell and fluid accumulation in the substantia propria of the conjunctiva. Frank vesicles may be seen in the conjunctiva[15,28] but they are not common. Primary keratopathy with punctate epitheliopathy in vesicles has also been reported [14,25,29-31] but this is also not common.

The chronic conjunctivitis may remit, sometimes for long periods, with eventual exacerbation and eventual development (usually within 3 to 4 years) of a similar, though asymmetric conjunctivitis in the opposite eye. Progression of the subepithelial fibrosis results first in a "shrinkage" of the conjunctiva, so that the normally deep fornices are foreshortened and, as the process continues, frank symblephara appear. Anatomy of the lid and adnexal components becomes deformed, disturbing the lid architecture and normal lid/globe relationship. The subepithelial fibrotic process alters the orientation of lash follicles, causing aberrant lash growth. There may even be enough fibrosis to produce cicatricial entropion.

Profound keratopathy can develop secondary to trichiasis and distichiasis, entropion, meibomianitis, tear insufficiency, and corneal exposure Corneal epitheliopathy, persistent epithelial defect, corneal stromal ulceration, and neovascularization may develop with astonishing rapidity. Secondary microbial keratitis is fairly common, and perforations of the cornea and endophthalmitis have been reported.[2,32,33] In the end the cornea is completely scarred, vascularized, and keratinized. Ankyloblepharon immobilizes the globe.

EXTRAOCULAR MANIFESTATIONS

Other sites affected by CP include skin, scalp, oral mucosa, nasal mucosa, pharynx, larynx, esophagus, vagina, urethra, and anus. A representative report of frequency of involvement of these various sites[27] appears in Table I.

Scarring of mucosa in nose and mouth is usually not debilitating, though the active mucosal ulcers in these areas during disease activity can be. The desquamative gingivitis present in nearly all patients with CP commonly results in bone loss and need for dental extractions. Scarring of the vaginal, urethral, and anal mucosa can produce progressive stricture formation, and the only known fatal consequences of CP are asphyxiation secondary to lodging of a food bolus in an esophageal stricture, and asphyxiation due to tracheal scarring and mucus accumulation.

The skin lesions which can occur in patients with CP may be of two types: recurrent vesiculobullous lesions similar to but smaller than those seen in bullous pemphigoid (these rupture and heal without significant scarring); and erythematous plaques of the head and neck that evolve into pruritic blisters which rupture and leave atrophic scars. This latter type of dermatitis has been called Brusting-Perry CP and it shares immunopathologic features with both pure mucosal CP and bullous pemphigoid of the skin, thereby placing it on the pemphigoid clinical spectrum.[34]

Hardy et al[27] reported ocular involvement in 62 of 81 cases of CP (76.5%). An average incidence of 66% is obtained when Hardy's cases are combined with the series of 30 CP cases published by Lever,[35] the 85 cases of Shklar and McCarthy,[36] and the 65 cases of Person and Rogers.[37]

HISTOLOGY AND IMMUNOPATHOLOGY

In 1953, Lever[3] demonstrated the histopathologic distinction between pemphigus and pemphigoid, thereby further subdividing the catholic view of blistering dermatoses. He documented that the central histopathologic feature in pemphigus is a loss of intercellular attachment bridges, with resultant detachment of cells from one another, or *acantholysis.* Thus bullae develop *within* the epidermis, with epidermal cells bordering the cavity of the bulla on all sides. Pemphigoid, on the other hand, is characterized by a separation of basal epithelium from underlying basement membrane, so that a *subepidermal* vacuole develops; this enlarges to produce a *subepidermal* bulla with no evidence of acantholysis.

The histopathologic characteristics of the conjunctiva in CP have been well described.[38-46] Squamous metaplasia of the epithelium, reduction in goblet cell numbers, infiltration of the substantia propria by chronic inflammatory cells (lymphocytes and plasma cells), and fibrosis of the substantia propria with new connective tissue formation are the predominant features. Occasional eosinophils and a few neutrophils have been described in some specimens.[46] Neutrophils are more abundant within and beneath the conjunctival epithelium during acute explosive episodes of the disease.[21]

The ultrastructural characteristics described by Carroll and Kuwabara[47] include epithelial derangement with extensive tonofibrils and desmosomes, epithelial basement membrane zone (BMZ) separation, fragmentation, and reduplication, and collagen fibril disorganization in the substantia propria.

The immunopathologic abnormalities of patients with CP are not restricted to the eye. Bean and colleagues[48] reported that 50% of their patients with ocular CP had elevated levels of serum IgA. Waltman and Yarian[49] found circulating autoantibodies, including antipancreas, thyroid, adrenal, and, most notably, antinuclear antibody (ANA) in 67% of patients with ocular CP. And 50% of CP patients can be shown during times of disease activity to have circulating autoantibody specific for epithelial and basement membrane.[50] Mondino et al[51] has reported a possible association of human leukocyte antigen (HLA)-B12 with CP. The essential criterion for establishing the diagnosis of CP affecting the eyes is the demonstration of immunoreactant deposition at the conjunctival BMZ.

The demonstration of immunoreactant deposition at the BMZ requires special care. Bean et al[48] reported that two of three conjunctival specimens from patients with suspected CP were positive by immunofluorescence (IF) techniques for IgG deposition at the BMZ. These two patients had classic CP activity elsewhere (skin and oral mucosa), with IgG deposition at the BMZ in these sites as well. The patient without BMZ immunoreactant deposition was the only one with disease activity limited to the eyes; this patient was not described, and one might question the diagnosis. One might also question Bean's assay sensitivity and his choice of antisera, which were directed against human IgG, IgA, IgM, and C_3, the third component of complement. For reasons that are as yet unclear, CP patients may show only IgE, IgD, C_4, or properdin factor B deposition at the conjunctival epithelial BMZ. One must, therefore, include antisera to these immunoreactants when performing immunopathologic analysis of conjunctiva from patients with suspected CP.

The avidin-biotin complex (ABC) immunoperoxidase technique, developed since Bean's studies, is approximately 1000 times more sensitive than IF and hence can detect BMZ immunoreactant deposition in considerably smaller amounts than previously possible. Though the ABC technique is more labor intensive than IF, it is an important addition to the diagnostic armamentarium in cases of suspected CP which are IF negative.

In earlier studies on immunoreactant deposition at the BMZ of conjunctiva from patients with suspected CP, Furey and colleagues[52] found 3 of 10 patients positive at the BMZ for IgG or IgA; Herron[53] demonstrated IgG at the BMZ of 1 patient, and Mondino et al[54] showed 8 of 12 patients to have IgA, IgG, and/or C_3 present at the BMZ of the conjunctiva.

We believe, given the improved antisera and high sensitivity of currently available immunopathologic techniques, that detection of immunoreactant deposition at the epithelial BMZ should be a requirement for diagnosis of CP. Appropriate control antisera can completely eliminate false positives (such as reported in cases of Mooren's ulcer and staphylococcal keratitis[55]). In our experience, even patients with extreme conjunctival inflammation due to other causes do not have linear deposition of immunoreactants at the epithelial BMZ. Immunoreactant deposition can occur at the skin epidermal BMZ and at the conjunctival epithelial BMZ in lupus erythematosus; but we know of no reports, nor have we ever observed a case, of lupus erythematosus that produced clinical ocular findings suggestive of CP.

TABLE I*: CUTANEOUS AND MUCOUS MEMBRANE INVOLVEMENT IN 81 CASES OF CP

SITE	NO OF PATIENTS
Mouth	68
Eyes	62
Pharynx	35
Nose	31
Larynx	24
Genitalia	
Female	18/52
Male	6/29
Skin	19
Anus	9
Esophagus	6

*From Hardy KM, et al: *Arch Dermatol* 1971; 104:467.

TABLE II: DIFFERENTIAL DIAGNOSIS OF CICATRIZING CONJUNCTIVITIS

CP
Trachoma
Corynebacterium diphtheriae conjunctivitis
Adenoviral conjunctivitis
Streptococcal conjunctivitis
Sarcoidosis
Progressive systemic sclerosis
Sjögren's syndrome
Practolol-induced conjunctivitis
Stevens-Johnson syndrome
Toxic epidermal necrolysis
Dermatitis herpetiformis
Epidermolysis bulbosa
Pemphigus vulgaris
Atopic blepharoconjunctivitis
Rosacea blepharoconjunctivitis
Prophyria cutanea tarda
Erythroderma ichthyosiform congenita
Conjunctival trauma

These immunopathologic features of CP are identical to those found in the skin of patients with bullous pemphigoid, and hence CP is considered by most investigators to be one of several pemphigoid-type disorders. One notable difference between bullous pemphigoid and CP is the presence in bullous pemphigoid of large amounts of circulating autoantibodies reactive with one or more components in basement membrane. Patients with active bullous pemphigoid usually have easily detectable (by indirect IF techniques) circulating autoantibodies to BMZ of some normal tissue substrate, such as monkey esophagus or guinea pig lip. CP patients rarely have such easily detectable autoantibodies. When such autoantibodies are found the titer is frequently quite low, and their demonstration usually depends on use of normal human mucous membrane (eg, conjunctiva) as substrate.

Only occasionally do patients with CP demonstrate circulating intercellular antibodies to epithelial substrates.[56] Two of the better immunopathologic CP studies performed in the recent past are those of Rogers and colleagues[57] and Laskaras and Angelopoulos.[58] Rogers and associates studied 23 patients with CP affecting the oral mucosa, and found a linear, continuous pattern of immunoreactant deposition at the BMZ in 83% of biopsy specimens. Complement studies provided data supportive of complement pathway activation in CP tissue, and deposition of IgA with factor B, properdin, and C_3 raised the possibility of alternative pathway activation. Laskaras and Angelopoulos[58] studied 33 patients with CP affecting the oral mucosa, and found a linear continuous pattern of immunoreactant deposition at the BMZ in 97% of the biopsy specimens. Circulating antibasement membrane antibodies were present in 36% of the patients in low titer (1:10 to 1:40) when normal oral mucosa was used as substrate. These authors emphasized that their studies further support the concept that CP and bullous pemphigoid represent variants of the same disease spectrum.

Finally, a number of other disorders and phenomena can cause chronic conjunctivitis and/or cicatricial changes (such as fornix foreshortening and/or symblepharon formation) that appear similar to many of the pathologic conjunctival changes seen in CP (Table II).

Some forms of infectious conjunctivitis (trachoma, adenovirus, *Corynebacterium diphtheriae*, and streptococcus) may cause conjunctival cicatrization. At least three systemic disorders with ocular manifestations may eventually produce fornix foreshortening (sarcoidosis, progressive systemic sclerosis, and Sjogren's syndrome). Chronic use of topical ocular drugs (epinephrine, echothiophate iodide, pilocarpine, and idoxyuridine) can be associated with conjunctival changes indistinguishable from CP (as we will discuss later). Certain skin and mucus membrane disorders may involve the conjunctiva and result in clinical signs indistinguishable from CP; practolol-induced eruption, Stevens-Johnson syndrome, toxic epidermal necrolysis, dermatitis herpetiformis, epidermolysis bullosa, pemphigus vulgaris, atopic skin disease with associated blepharokeratoconjunctivitis, rosacea blepharo-conjunctivitis prophyria cutanea tarda, and erythroderma ichthyo-siform congenita. Finally, ocular trauma due to chemical or thermal burn, or to multiple surgeries can produce conjunctival scarring similar to that seen in CP.

ASSOCIATED DISEASES

One accepted circumstantial criterion for considering a disease to probably be an autoimmune disorder is "guilt by association": association of the disease with other established autoimmune disorders. Currently available data are insufficient to warrant the conclusion that CP is associated with other autoimmune disorders. Although Spigel and Winkelmann[59] describe three patients with CP and rheumatoid arthritis or ankylosing spondylitis, they did not present their epidemiologic data regarding "at risk" and control populations, and therefore the paper must be considered simply an interesting case report. There is also a single case report of a patient with CP and systemic lupus erythematosus.[60] We specifically address this question of disease association later.

The question of CP association with internal malignancy is more provocative. Krain and Bierman[61] showed, after a decade of speculation about an association between blistering dermatosis and malignancy,[62] that pemphigus vulgaris and internal malignancies are causally related by accepted established epidemiologic criteria.[63]

Rook[64] reported one case of pemphigoid in a patient with carcinoma of the bronchus. Stone and Schroeter,[65] found no association with malignancy in their series of 73 patients with bullous pemphigoid, and Lim and associates[66] were unable to establish a relationship between pemphigoid and malignant disease in 103 patients. Greer and colleagues[67] reported on a patient with CP and metastatic carcinoma of the lung, and stated that the possible association of CP and malignancy had not been adequately studied; they suggested that a large series of patients with CP would have to be studied before conclusions could be drawn about this disease and cancer. We believe data to be presented later in this thesis will accomplish this goal.

TREATMENT

Several authors have noted that topical steroids and lubricants, traditionally used for the treatment of chronic cicatrizing conjunctivitis, are completely ineffective in controlling progression of CP. Periodic subconjunctival steroid injections can be temporally ameliorating, but are of no long-term benefit and eventually produce cataract.

High-dose systemic steroids can be effective therapy for CP, just as they care for bullous pemphigoid; they are, however, not uniformly successful in controlling CP activity. The long-term consequences of this therapy can be devastating. Hardy et al,[27] in a series of 81 patients with CP, found that the equivalent of 40 mg of prednisone per day was necessary to control disease progression. Despite this high dosage, 17 of 62 patients with ocular involvement became blind during treatment; 1 patient died from steroid-induced pneumonia; another had a severe gastrointestinal hemorrhage, and a third developed a brain hemorrhage with steroid-induced hypertension. Herron[53] used 80 mg of triamcinolone, tapering to a maintenance dose of 40 mg every other day. This regimen was successful in healing active mucosal ulcers in the subject of his single case report, but progression of symblepharon and corneal pannus was not halted.

Methotrexate,[68] azathioprine,[69] and cyclophosphamide[70] were eventually employed by investigators for the treatment of the life-threatening consequences of pemphigus vulgaris and for the morbidity associated with bullous pemphigoid. Investigators turned to the cytotoxic immunosuppressive drugs because circumstantial evidence implicated immunoregulatory dysfunction in these diseases and because the dangers of long-term prednisone therapy were unacceptable.

It was natural, therefore, that these drugs should also be employed in the treatment of CP. In 1974, Dave and Vickers[71] reported the results of therapy with azathioprine and prednisone in the treatment of four patients with CP. They had turned to this therapy because it worked so well in bullous pemphigoid and in pemphigus vulgaris, because CP immunopathology is very similar to that of bullous pemphigoid, and because long-term prednisone therapy carried unacceptable risks. Their initial patient had developed steroid-induced diabetes mellitus; and although the CP stabilized while the patient was receiving prednisone, it relapsed when the steroid was discontinued. The disease subsided once again when azathioprine was substituted for prednisone, and relapsed 1 year later when azathioprine dosage was tapered; the disease was once again controlled by increasing the azathioprine dosage. In their second patient who also had steroid-induced diabetes, CP was controlled with the addition of azathioprine and tapering of the systemic prednisone. In their third patient, CP could not be controlled by high doses of prednisone, but was controlled completely when azathioprine was added to the regimen. Azathioprine was discontinued 1 year after the disease had been controlled; the disease subsequently relapsed and was controlled once again with oral azathioprine therapy. Their fourth patient, whose disease was controlled by azathioprine therapy, suffered a relapse while still taking the drug. Brody and Pirozzi[72] reported on one case of a patient with CP whose severe, bilateral ocular involvement progressed in spite of steroid treatment. Subsequent azathioprine therapy also proved inadequate. The patient had severe eye, mouth, and esophageal involvement. The disease was controlled completely by 200 mg of cyclophosphamide/day; steroid was subsequently tapered and discontinued.

In 1953 Rook and Waddington[73] reported that 11 of 17 patients with bullous pemphigoid responded to treatment with sulfapyridine. Person and Rogers[74] confirmed these observations, and also noted the efficacy of dapsone, a drug previously used to treat leprosy and dermatitis herpetiformis. Rogers and associates[75] extended dapsone therapy to 24 patients with CP, 17 of whom had ocular involvement. Twelve of the 17 patients responded well, in that active conjunctival inflammation was substantially reduced; 4 patients developed dapsone intolerance that necessitated drug withdrawal.

EXPERIMENTAL STUDIES

STUDY PROCEDURE

Place and Dates of Study

Our systematic study and care of patients with ocular inflammatory disease began in July 1975. Like most efforts of this sort, the investigation has evolved and continues to evolve, both in terms of disease entities most intensely studied and in terms of procedures and study protocols. Thus, the 154 patients with CP affecting the eyes seen to date in the Immunology and Uveitis Unit have been evaluated and treated on our protocols to varying degrees. This report includes all patients, seen from July 1, 1975 until June 30, 1985 on whom we have adequate follow-up information, that is, the patients are under our care or we have current narrative and photographic follow-up information from the referring physician. This study group comprised 130 patients.

General Study Protocol

The general study protocol developed for our patients with CP is shown in Appendix I. In brief, we obtain a thorough ocular and medical history from each new patient and perform a complete ophthalmic examination; the findings are recorded on the data forms shown in Appendix II. We then obtain seven photographs of each eye. This standardized sequence of photographs has been performed identically, with the same photographic equipment and magnification parameters since the inception of these studies. The photographs are crucial to the successful operation of our program, since they often form the basis of our determination of whether progressive cicatrization has occurred or is occurring. The seven photographs are in primary gaze, gaze right, gaze left, up gaze (with lower lid gently pulled down, revealing the inferior fornix), down gaze (with upper lid retracted), upper tarsus (flipped upper lid), and lower tarsus (everted lower lid). This same sequence is repeated at every evaluation.

Patients are then sent to the laboratory for baseline blood and urine studies: white blood count with differential, hemoglobin, hematocrit platelets, erythrocyte sedimentation rate, glucose-6-phosphate dehydrogenase screen, autoantibody screen (for rheumatoid factor [RF] and ANA), and urinalysis. Serum is collected for determination of circulating autoantibodies to conjunctival epithelial basement membrane. HLA typing and serum screening (by Raji cell assay and C1q binding assay) for circulating immune complexes was done in a series of 30 patients (Appendix III).

Education

The patients then return to the Immunology and Uveitis Unit, after this rest from the initial ocular examination and photography. I then conduct an educational session, in which I describe to the patient the possible diagnoses, the usual natural history of CP, and our plan, should the patient choose to continue with us, for further studies and treatment. Patients are strongly advised to buy a portable tape recorder and bring it with them during each visit, so that they can review answers to questions and instructions regarding medication.

Study and Management

In a series of patients, we collected tears and mucus samples and conducted tear evaporation and impression cytology studies, then had the patients return 1 week later for conjunctival biopsy. The usual routine, however, was to obtain a biopsy specimen of bulbar conjunctiva as the next step after the education session. Two series of patients (3 in one and 10 in another) had inferior fornix and limbal bulbar conjunctival biopsy for histopathologic and immunopathologic analysis. In no instance were the fornix conjunctival biopsy positive for immunoreactant deposition at the BMZ and the bulbar conjunctival biopsy negative. Additional fornix foreshortening and symblepharon formation invariably resulted from fornix biopsies. We therefore changed our routine, and now perform bulbar conjunctival biopsy at the limbus in an area of clinical conjunctival inflammation. (A more complete description of biopsy technique and tissue handling is presented later.) Polysporin ointment is instilled into the biopsied eye and a pressure dressing is applied. The patient is instructed to change the dressing twice daily and to instill Polysporin ointment and dexamethasone phosphate (0.1%) ointment at each dressing change for 7 days. Questions are answered, educational handout material is dispensed, and an appointment is made for the patient to return in 2 weeks.

On the return visit the findings are reviewed, questions are answered, and recommendations for therapy are made. If the patient cannot be followed by me, we insist that the patient be in direct contact with an oncologist or hematologist, so that the patient will receive appropriate care and longitudinal monitoring while on chemotherapy. Referrals are made: for example, advanced gingival disease, a relatively common finding in patients with pemphigoid, requires appropriate dental care. Patients with symptoms even remotely suggestive of esophageal involvement are referred to a gastroenterologist for barium swallow x-rays and endoscopy, since patients with esophageal strictures may die from asphyxiation while attempting to swallow food. Therapy of confounding conditions, such as trichiasis, distichiasis, sicca syndrome, blepharitis, meibomianitis, and lagophthalmos is begun. Left untreated, these conditions produce conjunctival inflammation and irritation that make it impossible to determine whether increased levels of systemic chemotherapy are needed.

The following sections explain in more detail the treatment and elimination of these confounding variables, the development of our staging system, and the technique for biopsy and tissue analysis.

STUDY POPULATION

Demography

Our study population consisted of 130 patients with biopsy-proven CP affecting the eyes. The average age at onset was 64, with a range of 20 to 87 years. Twenty-three patients were younger than 60; 6 were under the age of 40. The mean duration of ocular involvement at the time of our first evaluation was 2.8 years, with a range of 1 to 11 years. Sixty-four percent of the patients were women (ratio, 7/4). Only four patients were nonwhite, but since the patient population referred to our hospital is predominantly white, we cannot conclude that this finding suggests any racial predilection for CP.

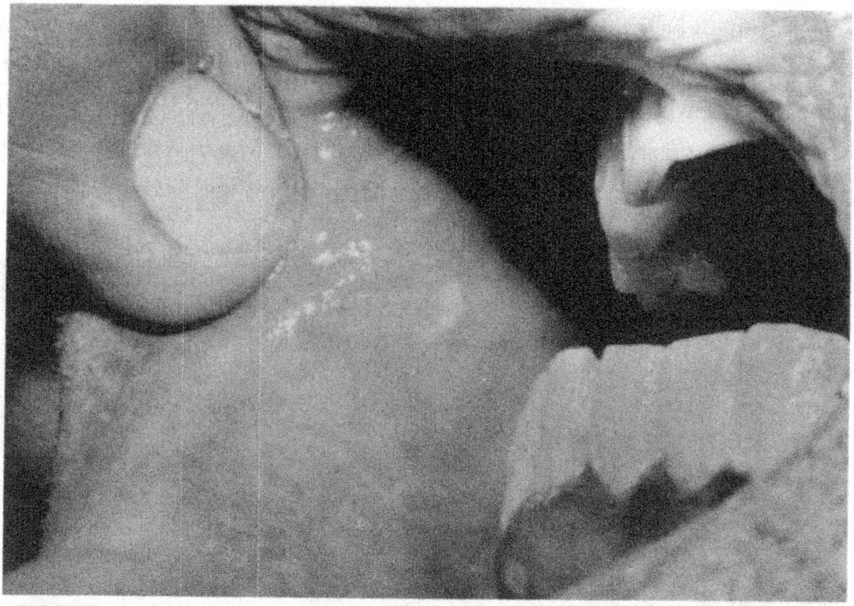

FIGURE 1: Vertically oval active buccal mucosal ulcer. Note also inflamed gingiva.

Clinical Characteristics

The sites of involvement of mucous membranes are shown in Table III. Obviously, because of the nature of our selection process, the eye was involved in all patients. The most common extraocular site of involvement was buccal (Fig 1) and pharyngeal mucosa. Note, however, that the number of patients with esophageal involvement (12) was not trivial; 2 of those patients experienced nearly fatal asphyxiation necessitating emergency tracheostomies because of food bolus entrapment at a stricture point. Esophageal involvement was usually "silent" in that little or no pain was associated with the esophageal lesions until esophageal strictures sufficient to impede comfortable passage of food developed. Vaginal involvement was also frequently "silent," especially in older women, and I suspect our figure of 5 cases of vaginal involvement in 83 women is an underestimate of its true frequency. I also wonder about involvement of sinus mucosa in CP; many of our patients complained of sinus congestion and excess sinus mucus discharge prior to successful control of the disease through chemotherapy. Chronic "gingivitis" is extremely common in this disease (Fig 2). It is an often-overlooked manifestation. Appropriate dental care is an important component in the overall program of therapy for patients with CP. The skin lesions noted in the 10% of our CP patients were not bullae or vesicles, but rather were the Brusting-Perry type lesions (erythematous plaques), most frequently found on the scalp (Fig 3).

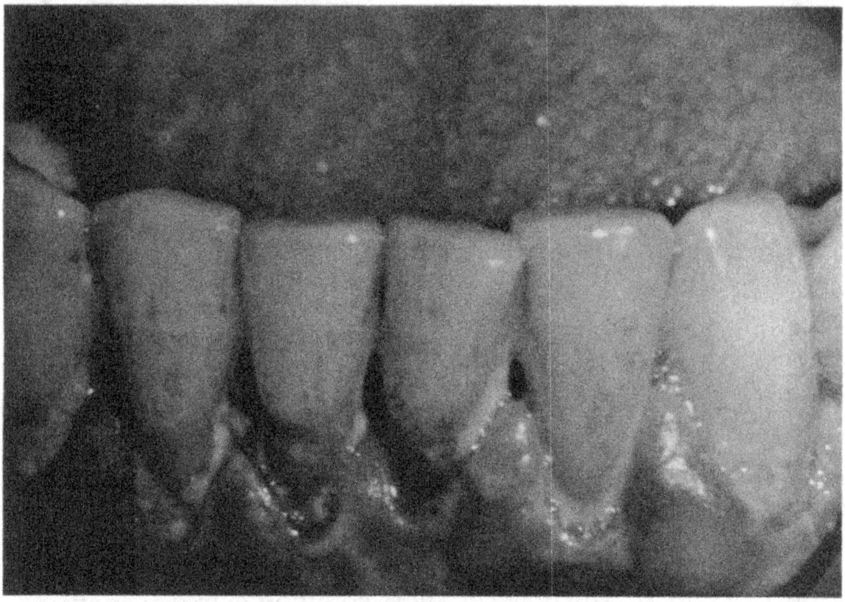

FIGURE 2: Chronic gingivitis, with resultant bone resorption and periodontal disease which will necessitate extraction of multiple teeth.

Table III also shows the site of onset for the 130 patients. The most common onset (and presenting diagnosis) was chronic unilateral conjunctivitis.

Our staging system is described later. Most patients (86%) had at least stage III disease, usually (91%) bilaterally, when we first saw them. Forty percent had keratopathy sufficient to reduce vision to 20/200 or worse in at least one eye (Table IV).

Associated Diseases

Associated systemic autoimmune diseases were present in 23 patients; 19 had rheumatoid arthritis, 3 had systemic lupus erythematosus, and 1 patient, to be described in detail below, had multiple autoimmune phenomena. This frequency of autoimmune disease (17.7%) is significantly higher than the expected frequency (4%) in a population of 130 patients in the age range 20 to 90 years ($P < 0.01$).

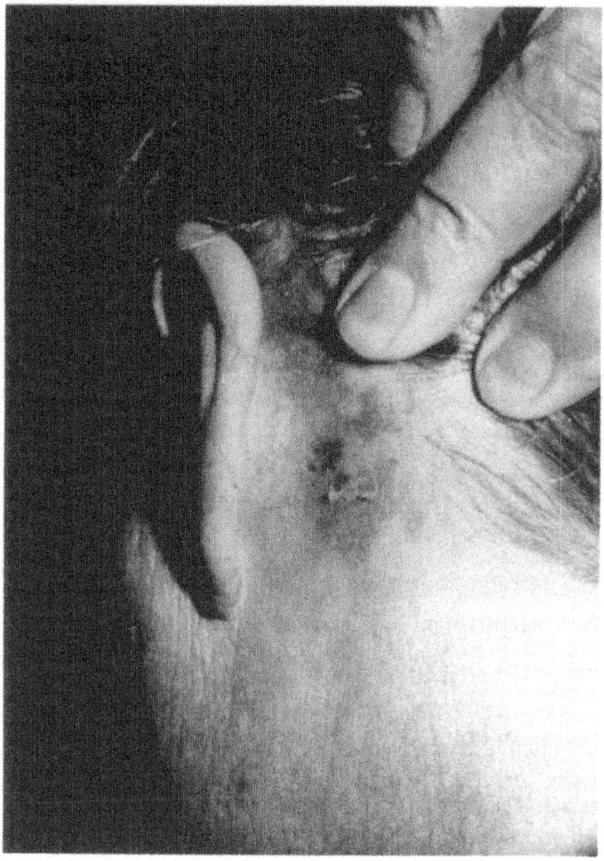

FIGURE 3: Brusting-Percy CP dermatitis. These ulcers will heal with scar formation.

Seven patients in this study population developed or had had cancer of some type. Carcinoma of the bladder and breast each occurred in two patients; adenocarcinoma of the lung, squamous carcinoma of the tongue, and bone cancer (spine) each occurred in one patient. This incidence of malignancy (5%) is not different from the norm; the chance of developing a malignancy during one's life from age 20 to 90 years is approximately 25% for men (slightly higher for women). These data, then, do not suggest an association between CP and malignancy.

TABLE III: SITES OF INVOLVEMENT AND ONSET IN 130 CASES OF CP AFFECTING THE EYES

SITE	NO. OF PATIENTS	
	INVOLVEMENT	ONSET
Eyes	130	106
Mouth	19	7
Pharynx	9	0
Nose	15	9
Larynx	5	0
Esophagus	12	0
Urethra	4	0
Vagina	5	0
Anus	8	0
Skin	12	8

TABLE IV: DEGREE OF OCULAR INVOLVEMENT IN 130 CASES OF CP

STAGE*				BILATERAL	KERATOPATHY†	VISUAL ACUITY ≤ 20/200	
I	II	III	IV			ONE EYE	BOTH EYES
6	13	99	12	118	52	52	18

*Most advanced eye.
†More profound than simple SPK: erosions, scars, vascularization, ulcer.

Only one of the patients (with bladder cancer) was receiving cytotoxic therapy (azathioprine) at the time his malignancy was diagnosed; all others had been diagnosed and treated for cancer previously. The patient who developed squamous carcinoma of the tongue had prednisone but no cytotoxic therapy before development of the carcinoma; he died within 8 months of the diagnosis of the cancer.

STAGING SYSTEM

Our staging system, like Mondino and Brown's,[22] is based on conjunctival changes. Their staging system relies on the amount of conjunctival shrinkage or fornix foreshortening: stage I, 0% to 25% loss of conjunctival fornix; stage II, 25% to 50% loss; stage III, approximately 75% loss; and stage IV is end stage disease, with total fornix obliteration and keratinization.

We defined stage I as the presence of chronic conjunctivitis with subepithelial fibrosis, best seen as white bands in the upper and lower tarsal conjunctiva (Fig 4A and B). Stage II is characterized by inferior fornix fore-shortening (Fig 5). Stage III is defined by the appearance of a symblepharon (Fig 6).

Patients in this stage also show a wide range of pathologic changes that include varying degrees of keratopathy, corneal neovascularization, trichiasis, distichiasis, and tear insufficiency. Stage IV is end stage disease, with ankyloblepharon, severe sicca syndrome, and extreme ocular surface keratinization (Fig 7).

Other staging systems may be equally or more useful in describing and in managing CP affecting the eyes, but ours has served us well, providing a useful framework for decisions concerning therapy (see Clinical Trials). Although other pathologic changes such as trichiasis, distichiasis, entropion, meibomianitis, keratopathy, corneal neovascularization, and tear insufficiency are extremely important and must be carefully documented, we find progression from one stage to another, as described above, to be the best indicator of disease control or progression.

INDIVIDUAL STUDY PROTOCOLS AND RESULTS

Physiologic Studies

Tear Production—CP affecting the eyes has been called a dry-eye syndrome.[76] Although the disease does cause tear insufficiency and, in stage IV, nearly total xerosis of the ocular surface, we have been impressed by the volume of tear fluid present in most patients with CP, even well into stage III. We therefore measured tear production with a modification of Schirmer's test.[77] Briefly, the relationship between fluid volume and Schirmer strip wetting was studied by applying increasing amounts of normal saline solution to strips of Schirmer paper with a 5 μl syringe. The amount of wetting was measured for five separate determinations, and measurements were averaged for each microliter of fluid. Results were analyzed by the method of least squares, and a correlation coefficient was computed. The effect of topical anesthetic on the conjunctiva was demonstrated by the use of a Cochet-Bonnet anesthesimeter in ten normal adults (20 eyes) who ranged in age from 20 to 40 years. Measurements were obtained from inferotemporal and nasal conjunctiva and from cornea, before and after instillation of 50 μl of 0.5% proparacaine hydrochloride. Data were plotted and analyzed for significance by the Student's *t*-test.

Schirmer strip wetting, both before and after instillation of topical anesthetic, and measurement of tear meniscus height were determined in normal volunteers. Persons who received ocular or systemic medication were excluded from the study, as were those with ocular disease or a history of ocular surgery within the previous 6 months. Study samples from two populations were used: group 1 consisted of 43 employees of our hospital (22 men and 21 women) who ranged in age from 21 to 84 years; group 2 consisted of 190 persons, members (and their dependents) of the US Army (122 men and 68 women) from Ft Dix, NJ, who ranged in age from 12 to 80 years. Among both groups of patients, 40% ranged in age from 10 to 29 years, 28% from 30 to 49 years, 29% from 50 to 69 years, and 2% were more than 70 years. Thus, the study population was weighted toward the younger age groups. Schirmer strip wetting, with and without topical anesthetic, and measurement of tear meniscus height were determined for all persons in group 1; in group 2, Schirmer tests were conducted only after instillation of topical anesthetic in 102 persons, and both before and after anesthesia in 88 persons. The subjects' eyes were open during the test. All Schirmer tests were done with prepackaged, standardized, sterile strips of filter paper. Strips were placed over the lateral third of the lower lid, and results were determined after 5 minutes. In those volunteers who were given anesthetic, 50 µl of proparacaine hydrochloride was placed in each eye; after 1 minute, the cul-de-sac was gently blotted dry with a tissue. The mean, standard deviation, and standard error of the mean were determined separately for each group and were found to be similar; therefore, the data were combined for final analysis. The Student's *t*-test was used to determine the significance level of differences between mean values obtained in the study group.

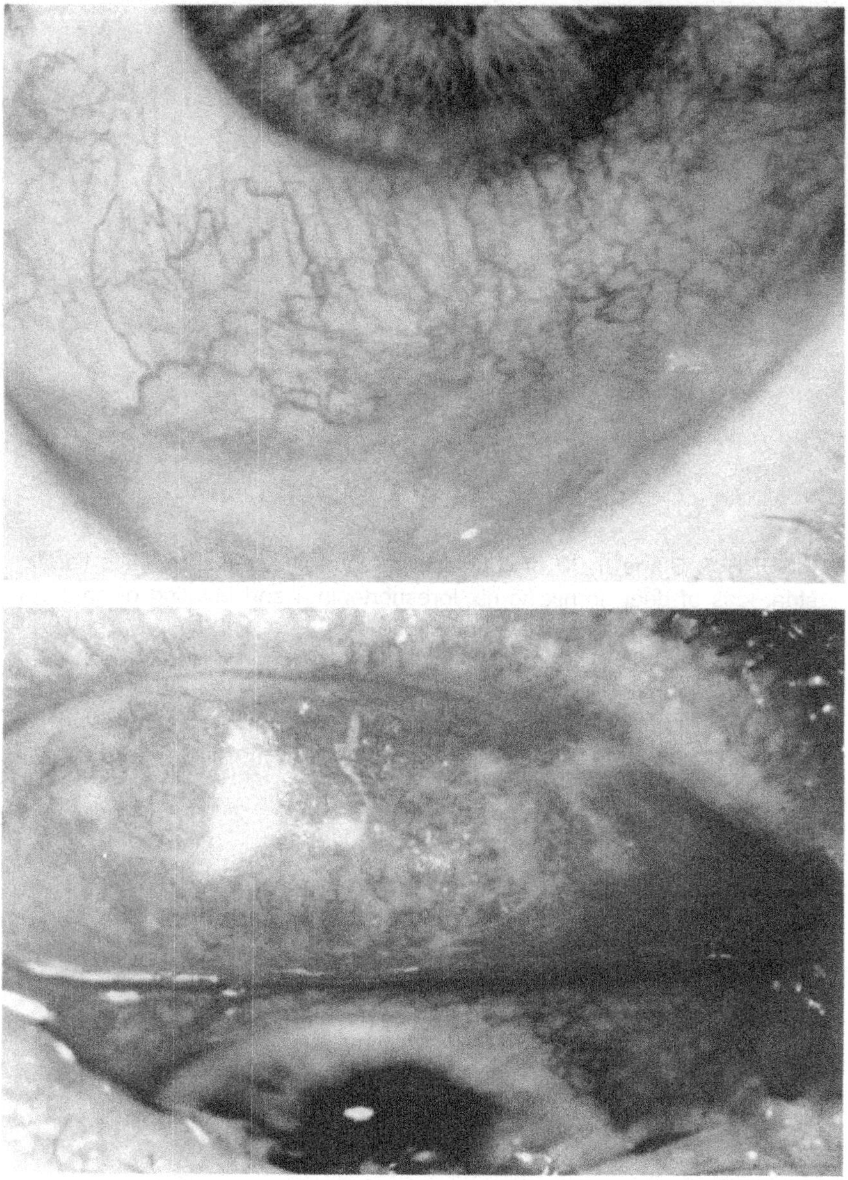

FIGURE 4: Stage I CP changes of conjunctiva. Note tarsal subepithelial white stria and, temporally, formation of "felt-work" subepithelial fibrosis in this case of chronic conjunctivitis secondary to CP. b: Similar tarsal subepithelial fibrotic changes in upper tarsus. These changes are very often overlooked in superior tarsus, and are very often present in stage I CP.

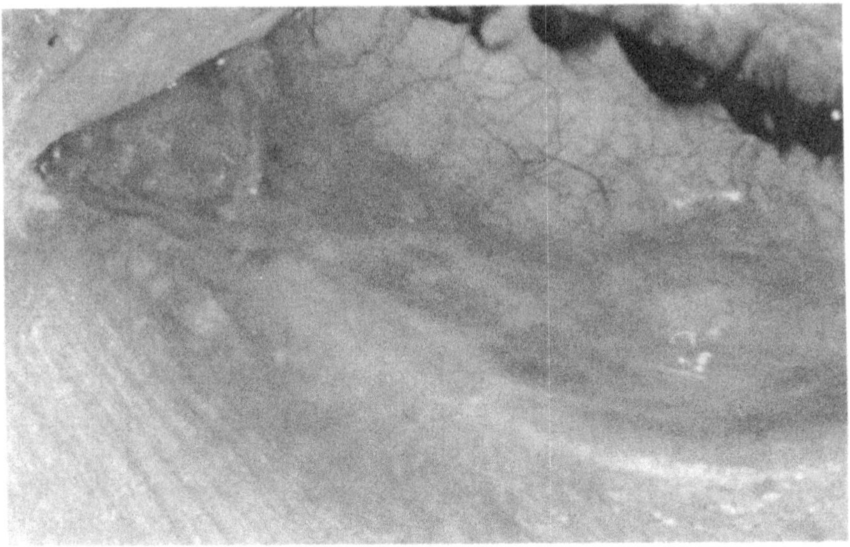

FIGURE 5: Stage II CP of conjunctiva. Note, in addition to white fibrotic stria, loss of deep fornix (fornix foreshortening) and blunting of angle of reflection of fornix conjunctiva onto globe.

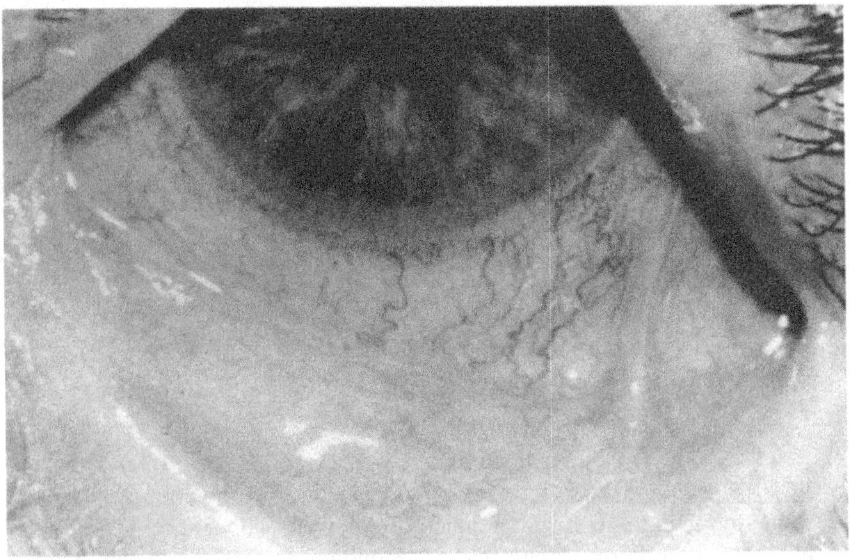

FIGURE 6: Stage III CP conjunctiva. In addition to extensive "felt-work" of subepithelial fibrosis, and fornix foreshortening, there is now frank symblepharon present temporally, most easily seen with lower lid retracted and patient gazing upwards.

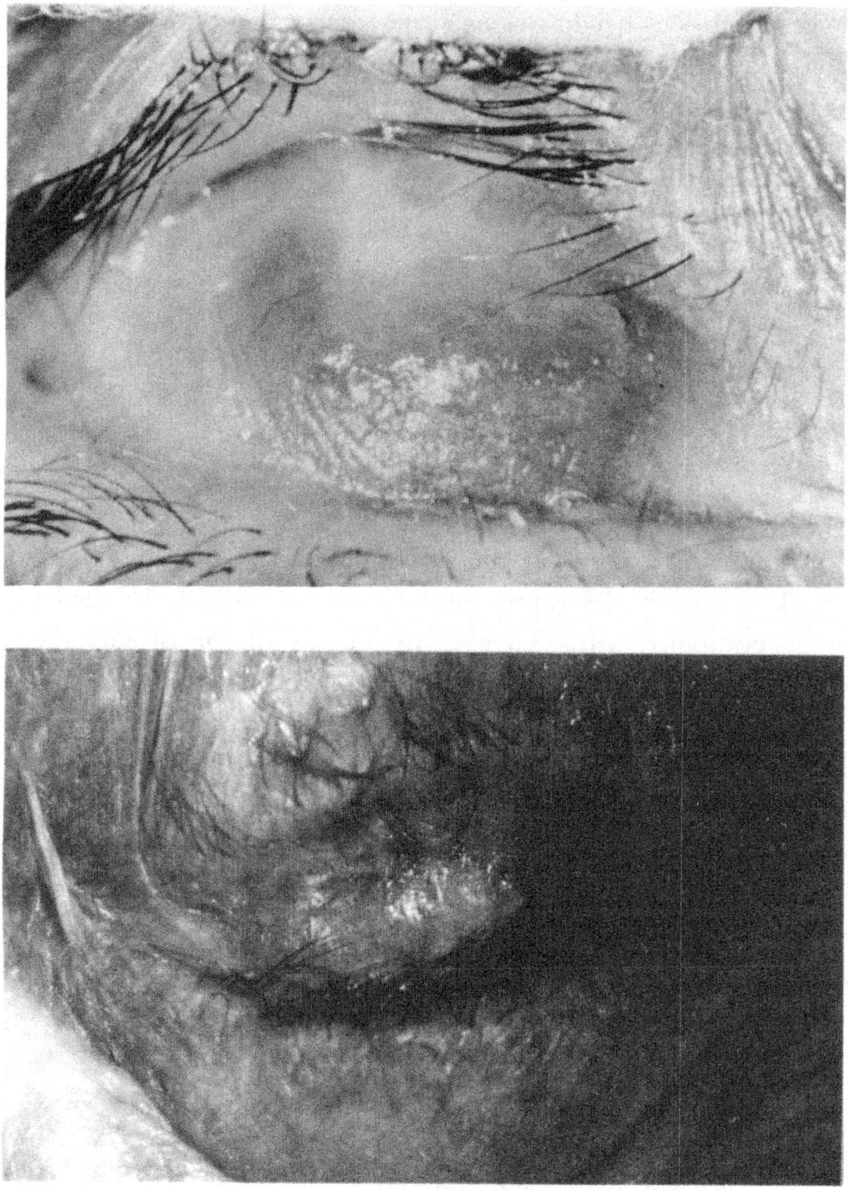

FIGURE 7: a: Stage IV CP affecting eyes. Anklyoblepharon has developed. Total xerosis has developed, and ocular surface epithelium is completely keratinized. b: Stage IV CP, with total ankyloblepharon and surface keratinization. Ocular surface is now skin-like.

Tear meniscus height was determined only in group 1. Prior to any manipulation of the eye, measurements were read from a reticule that was inserted into the eyepiece of a slit lamp. The reticule was calibrated so that actual readings, in 0.1-mm increments, could be made with 6x ocular. A distribution curve for meniscus height was plotted, and correlation coefficients were determined for meniscus height and Schirmer testing with and without topical anesthetic.

The relationship between the volume of fluid that was applied to the end of a Schirmer strip and the amount of wetting that was subsequently measured was precisely linear. The straight line, fitted to the data points by the least squares method, had a correlation coefficient of 0.98.

The difference in anesthesimeter values that were obtained in ten normal volunteers (20 eyes) before and after 0.5% proparacaine hydrochloride was instilled was profound. When the values for groups 1 and 2 were combined without regard to the sex or age of subjects, the mean Schirmer test value without anesthesia was 19.6 mm; for test with anesthesia, the mean was 11.9 mm. This represents a 40% mean reduction in wetting, a highly significant difference ($P < 0.001$), after the use of topical anesthetic.

A decrease in tear production with advancing age was not detected. When all men and women were compared without regard to age, no significant difference was found with respect to the sex of the individual in wetting of the Schirmer strip ($P < 0.1$).

Physicians who use topical anesthetic and blotting of the cul-de-sac as part of the Schirmer test procedure should accept a lower limit of normal than previously reported values. If Van Bijsterveld's value of 5.5 mm of wetting is taken as a cutoff point, 28% of normal men and 20% of normal women will be misclassified. If Schirmer's original value of 15 mm wetting is used as a cutoff value, results from 80% of normal men and 63% of normal women will be abnormal when anesthetic is used. Specificity improves if 3 mm or less is considered to be the cutoff point, since only about 15% of the population would normally be expected to show this small amount of wetting.

The results of our initial Schirmer analysis of 20 patients with active CP affecting the eyes are shown in Table V. Notice that stage III eyes do not differ from normal values.

Three repeat analyses (Table V) made after correction of trichiasis, entropion, and other confounding, irritating conditions demonstrated a reduction in Schirmer values, but the data clearly demonstrate that dramatic reduction in tear fluid volume is a late phenomenon in this disease. It presumably occurs as a result of obliteration of the lacrimal ducts by scarring, since no abnormality of the lacrimal gland itself has been documented. Tear volume deficiency is not an early, primary component in CP.

Tear Breakup Time—Tear breakup time (BUT) is defined as the interval between a complete blink and the appearance of the first randomly distributed dry spot on the cornea.[78] It has been emphasized that the random distribution of these spots is important, since it is well known that alterations in the epithelial surface will result in rapid breakup in the tear film.[79] If the dry spot consistently develops in one area, it is probably due to local factors and cannot be regarded as a true indication of BUT. The BUT is meant to be a measure of tear film stability per se and not a measure of ocular surface pathology responsible for an abnormal relationship between the tear film and the ocular surface.

We measured BUT in 20 patients with CP affecting the eyes after elimination of aberrant lashes. We employed the method of Lemp. Briefly, a slightly moistened fluorescein strip was applied to the inferior temporal bulbar conjunctiva, and the patient was asked to blink several times. The tear film was then scanned by slit lamp biomicroscopy with blue light while the patient gazed straight ahead without blinking. The time to appearance of the first dry spot was recorded five times in succession for each eye, and the average value was recorded as the BUT for that eye. Results from normal control patients confirmed Lemp's observations that a normal BUT is always greater than 10 seconds.

TABLE V: MEAN SCHIRMER VALUES AFTER TOPICAL ANESTHETIC IN 20 PATIENTS WITH STAGE III CP AFFECTING THE EYES

EYE	MEAN SCHIRMER VALUE (mm)	
	IRRITATING FACTORS PRESENT	IRRITATING FACTORS CORRECTED
OD	12 ± 3	8 ± 2
OS	10 ± 2	5 ± 2

TABLE VI: TER IN 8 PATIENTS WITH OCULAR CP

PATIENT	EYE	TER (gm/cm²/sec)
1	OD	36.7
	OS	23.0
2	OD	ND
	OS	15.1
3	OD	ND
	OS	26.7
4	OD	10.2
	OS	18.7
5	OD	19.7
	OS	31.0
6	OD	11.0
	OS	16.7
7	OD	25.2
	OS	—
8	OD	23.4
	OS	—
Mean TER		21.45
SD		± 2.27

TABLE VII: TEAR OSMOLARITY IN 8 PATIENTS WITH CP

PATIENT	EYE	TEAR OSMOLARITY (mOsm/l)
1	OD	317
	OS	309
2	OD	—
	OS	309
3	OD	310
	OS	312
4	OD	320
	OS	326
5	OD	304
	OS	300
6	OD	329
	OS	311
7	OD	307
	OS	317
8	OD	312
	OS	299
Mean		312.13
SD		± 2.21

The mean BUT in our CP patients was 5.3 ± 2.0 seconds before treatment and 10.4 ± 2.2 seconds after successful treatment with systemic chemotherapy. The pretreatment values could lead one to conclude that CP is a disease characterized by an abnormality of the preocular tear film.[80] As we will show below, however, this is an unwarranted conclusion since: (1) these eyes are not dry; (2) these eyes are not mucin-deficient; (3) there are alterations of the surface epithelium which make the value of BUT in assessing the tear film questionable; and (4) there are mucus deposits on the ocular surface of CP patients, and these deposits also undoubtedly markedly alter the dynamic relationship between the ocular surface and the preocular tear film.

Tear Evaporation Rate—In collaboration with Drs Miguel Refojo, Kenneth R. Kenyon, and Shaeffer Tseng, we measured the tear evaporation rate (TER) from eight patients with active CP affecting the conjunctiva. Briefly, swimming goggles, sealed with petroleum jelly, were worn by the study subject. A probe in the goggles allowed measurement of relative humidity. The subject was asked to open his eyes and to refrain from blinking for 60 seconds. The increased relative humidity due to evaporation from the tears was then determined.

As shown in Table VI the mean TER for these patients was 21.45 $\pm$ 2.27 X 10^{-7} gm/cm^2/sec, with a range of 10.2 to 36.7. The normal mean is 4.07 X 10^{-7} gm/cm^2/sec. Student's *t*-test for significance of difference between the TER for CP patients compared to normal individuals shows a significantly increased evaporation rate for CP patients ($P < 0.005$).

This increased TER could be the result of several different factors or combination of factors. Increased ocular temperature from the vascular dilatation associated with inflammation could facilitate evaporation. An abnormal lipid component of the preocular tear film, resulting from the "meibomianitis" so common in CP patients, could facilitate evaporation. And a preocular tear film of substantially different composition from normal (because of protein, inflammatory mediator, cellular debris, mucus, etc, content) might affect TER. It has been speculated that an abnormal ocular surface per se would increase the TER. This is unlikely, given the forces governing evaporation (surface area, temperature, vapor pressures). I suspect the increased TER seen in our CP patients results, in large measure, from an increased ocular surface temperature and from a decreased effective lipid layer on the surface of the preocular tear film. Studies are currently in progress in our laboratory to investigate these possibilities.

Tear Osmolarity—Osmolarity determinations were also performed, in collaboration with Dr Jeffrey Gilbard, on eight patients. Briefly, 0.2-ml tear samples were harvested by capillary action with 0.2-mm glass capillary tubes touching the tear meniscus. The samples were blown into a second capillary tube below a 1-cm column of immersion oil. The tear samples were later rescued with a fine-tipped capillary tube, and the osmolarity of each sample was determined via freezing point depression by use of a commercially available osmometer capable of measurements on samples as small as 0.1 ml with an accuracy of ± 0.76%.

The data are shown in Table VII. The mean tear osmolarity for these patients with CP was 312.13 ± 2.21 mOsm/l. Compared to tear osmolarity of 304 ± 10.4 mOsm/1 for normal individuals, this is not a statistically significant difference ($P > 0.05$).

Conjunctival Epithelial Mitotic Rate—We reported, at the 1984 ARVO meetings, that patients with CP exhibit hypermitotic activity of the conjunctival basal epithelium.[81]

The method employed for this study involved incubation of a 2-mm^2 piece of conjunctiva incubated immediately upon biopsy (always performed between 10:00 A.M. and noon to avoid diurnal variation effects) in Dulbecco's minimum essential medium, serum-free, with 10 µCi/ml, tritiated thymidine (New England Nuclear) at 37°C in a 5% $C0_2$-95% air tissue culture incubator for 2½ hours. A medium exchange to isotope free-medium is followed by a further incubation for ½ hour, and subsequent tissue fixation overnight in 10% buffered formalin. The tissue is then embedded in paraffin, sectioned at 7 µm, with subsequent section deparaffinization, and staining with periodic acid-Schiff (PAS), hematoxylin and eosin (H&E), and Giemsa stains. Unstained sections are dipped to insure removal of all excess paraffin. The slides are then dipped in Kodak NTB2 emulsion twice in total darkness, after warming the emulsion to 45°C. Slides are dried for 1 hour in total darkness and are stored in a light-tight box for 2 weeks at -20°C. Slides are developed in total darkness with Kodak D19, diluted 1:1 with water, 5-minute incubation at 18°C, followed by a tap water rinse, fixation with Kodak fixer at 18°C for 5 minutes, and subsequent washing in tap water.

Light microscopy is then performed to determine the number of tritiated thymidine-labeled cells (5-phase cells) in the autoradiographs. Such labeled cells are counted and the mitotic rate expressed as the number of labeled cells per 100 basal epithelial cells. A minimum of 200 basal cells are counted, and each specimen is counted by two observers in masked fashion. The results are shown in Table VIII.

The normal mitotic rate for conjunctival epithelium, as determined by this technique, is 1.68 ± 0.018/100 basal epithelial cells.[81] We measure, therefore, a fourfold increase above normal mitotic rate in patients with active CP, a strikingly significant increase ($P < 0.005$).

TABLE VIII: BASAL EPITHELIAL MITOTIC RATE IN CONJUNCTIVA FROM 10 PATIENTS WITH ACTIVE CP

CASE	MITOTIC RATE (LABELED CELLS/100 BASAL CELLS)
1	4.7
2	7.4
3	8.3
4	7.1
5	8.8
6	18.2
7	·4.8
8	3.8
9	8.8
10	4.0
Mean	7.59
SD	± 1.33

The mitotic rate did not vary with location. The normal mitotic rate of the human conjunctival epithelium was 1.68 labeled cells per 100 basal epithelial cells, a value comparable to that reported for the corneal epithelial mitotic rate in several animals and for some surface epithelia (ie, oral mucosa).

Changes in mitotic rate are observed under many circumstances. For example, tumors typically have increased mitotic rates, and the degree of increase of the mitotic rate has been used with various degrees of success as an indicator of malignancy. Increased mitotic rates are also typical responses of tissue to stress. Thus, the mitotic rate in bone marrow and thymus increases after trauma and antigenic stimulation. Similarly, epithelial tissues become hypermitotic in response to chemical or mechanical irritation, antigenic stimulus, or underlying inflammation.

Thoft and associates[81] have speculated that hypermitosis of the epithelium may not be a consequence of the conjunctival inflammation but may actually induce some of the clinical manifestations of the disease. There is no convincing evidence for this, and we now have accumulated substantial evidence supporting the classical concept of inflammation creating the pathologic changes.

MORPHOLOGY

Histopathology

Light Microscopy—Bulbar conjunctival biopsies were obtained from all 130 patients in our study group. One drop of 0.5% proparacaine hydrochloride is used for surface anesthesia, and 0.2 ml of 1% xylocaine was injected subconjunctivally 5 mm from the limbus in an area of clinically apparent conjunctival inflammation. Thirty to 60 seconds were allowed for spread of the injected anesthetic to the corneoscleral limbus. A 2-mm limbal peritomy was then created with Vannas scissors, and two radial relaxing incisions were extended 3 mm posteriorly. Subconjunctival tissue was undermined to bare sclera, and a flap of tissue was excised and divided for fixation and for cryostat processing.

The specimen for histopathologic analysis by light microscopy was placed in Karnovsky's fixative (1% paraformaldehyde, 1.25% glutaraldehyde, in 0.2 mol/l sodium cacodylate buffer). After overnight fixation, the specimen was transferred to 0.2 mol/l sodium cacodylate buffer, which was changed at least three times with buffer at 20-minute intervals. The specimen was then dehydrated through ascending concentrations of ethanol (50%, 70%, 95%, 100%), with three changes of each concentration at 20-minute intervals. The tissue specimen was infiltrated with glycol methacrylate solution overnight, and then embedded in the resin (Historesin, LKB-Produkter AB, Bromma, Sweden) and sectioned at 2 μm on a Sorvall JB-4 microtome. Sections were then stained with alkaline Giemsa, PAS, and H&E stains. Light microscopy was performed, and data for each specimen recorded on a standardized data recording sheet (Appendix IV). Three high-dry (500 X) fields were viewed; the numbers of epithelial goblet cells and the various inflammatory cell types in the substantia propria were counted. Table IX is a presentation of the results of light microscopy analyses of a representative sample of 30 of our 130 subjects.

Space requirements for presentation of all 130 specimens is prohibitive, but Table X is a summary of mean values obtained for the various histopathologic features from all 130 patients.

This histopathologic analysis of the 130 specimens produced several findings that had previously been unreported or that differ somewhat from earlier reports. The finding of epithelial metaplasia, of course, was expected (Figs 8 and 9). Somewhat unexpected, and different from previous reports, was the wide spectrum of epithelial morphology observed in specimens from patients with identical clinical findings (stage of disease, degree of conjunctival clinical inflammatory signs, Schirmer values, etc) (Fig 10). The large number of specimens analyzed in our study allowed us to see that the conjunctival morphology of patients with CP is abnormal but dynamic. It is a misconception, ie, that all patients with CP lack goblet cells; these goblet cells are often present (and may sometimes be plentiful) in patients with rather advanced stage III disease (Fig 11). As will be shown later, the conjunctival epithelial morphology in CP can be changed by systemic chemotherapy. Our studies of conjunctival biopsy specimens taken after achievement of disease quiescence showed that goblet cells had returned and squamous metaplastic changes had reverted toward normal.

The cellular infiltrate in the substantia propria is variable in cell density and in relative proportions of the various cell types. We were unable to correlate cell type predominance with degree of difficulty in achieving control through use of dapsone and/or other chemotherapeutic agents. The cellular density was, in all cases, greater than that in normal conjunctiva (Fig 12), and in many instances the cellular infiltrate was extreme (Fig 13). As will be seen below, the inflammatory cells in CP conjunctiva are metabolically highly active.

We found previously unreported vascular involvement in CP conjunctiva. Light microscopy revealed clear-cut vasculopathy with perivascular inflammatory cell infiltration in 20% of our specimens (Fig 14a and b). Ultrastructural studies, discussed below, showed that vasculopathy is the rule rather than the exception.

TABLE IX: LIGHT MICROSCOPY HISTOPATHOLOGY RESULTS

CASE	EPITHELIUM			SUBSTANTIA PROPRIA					PERIVASCULITIS
	SQUAMOUS METAPLASIA	GOBLET CELLS	PLASMA CELLS	LYMPHOCYTES	HISTIOCYTES	MAST CELLS	EOSINOPHILS	NEUTROPHILS	
1	Extreme	0	32	14	12	8	0	0	−
2	Mild	1	18	28	11	8	0	0	+
3	Moderate	1	24	10	8	9	0	0	−
4	Moderate	2	33	21	18	9	0	0	+
5	—	3	9	8	7	6	0	0	−
6	Extreme	0	10	14	8	5	0	0	−
7	Extreme	0	25	14	6	6	0	0	−
8	Moderate	0	27	17	10	6	0	1	−
9	Extreme	0	40	32	28	5	0	0	−
10	—	3	18	4	8	9	0	0	−
11	Mild	3	24	16	4	9	0	0	−
12	Extreme	0	12	20	12	6	0	0	+
13	Moderate	0	12	12	8	9	0	0	+
14	Mild	2	13	25	4	5	0	0	−
15	Moderate	0	14	18	7	6	0	0	−
16	—	3	12	12	6	8	0	0	+
17	Mild	2	20	6	4	9	1	0	−
18	Moderate	0	14	7	5	6	0	1	−
19	Moderate	0	17	9	7	5	0	0	−
20	Extreme	0	7	5	3	7	0	0	−
21	Extreme	0	16	11	9	9	1	0	−
22	Extreme	0	28	3	12	8	0	0	−
23	Extreme	0	5	8	7	5	0	0	−
24	Moderate	0	14	13	5	9	1	1	+
25	Moderate	1	18	16	4	4	0	0	−
26	Extreme	0	12	23	5	3	0	0	−
27	Extreme	0	25	17	9	5	0	0	−
28	Moderate	0	14	17	5	3	0	0	−
29	Mild	1	9	8	6	7	0	0	−
30	Mild	2	30	13	4	3	0	0	−

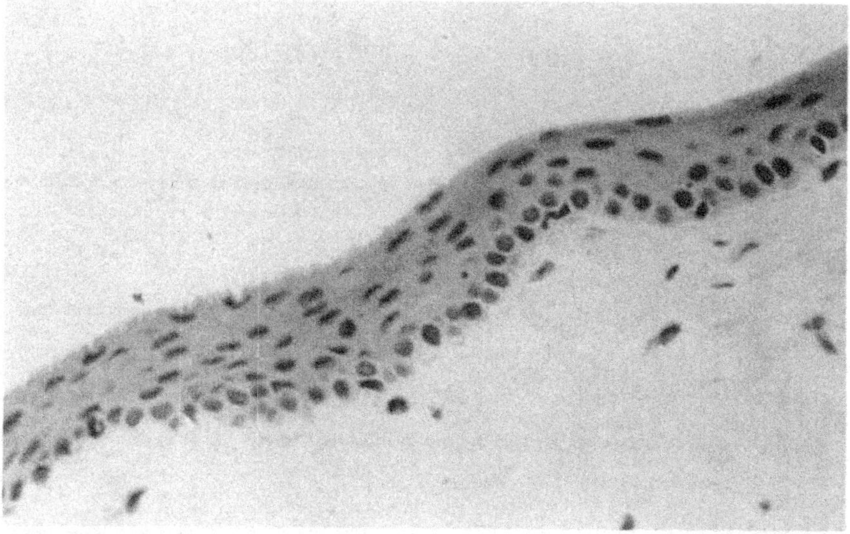

<u>FIGURE 8:</u> Normal human conjunctiva (H&E stain, X 400). Note nonkeratinized, squamous epithelium, approximately five layers thick, with small numbers of resident mononuclear cells in underlying substantia propria.

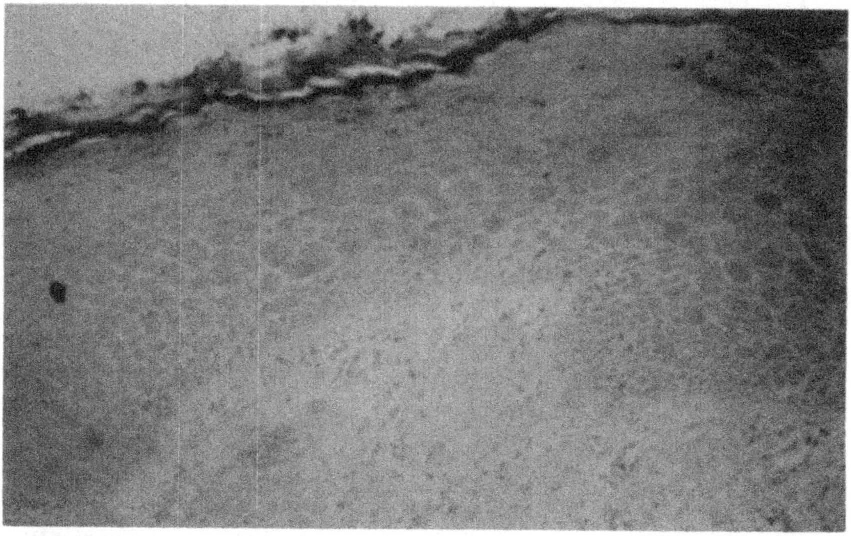

<u>FIGURE 9:</u> CP conjunctiva (acridine/orange oil red O stain, x 400). Note squamous metaplasia, with stratified squamous epithelium, thickening of epithelial layer, and presence of "prekeratin" as disclosed by reddish-orange stain of most superficial layer of epithelial cells.

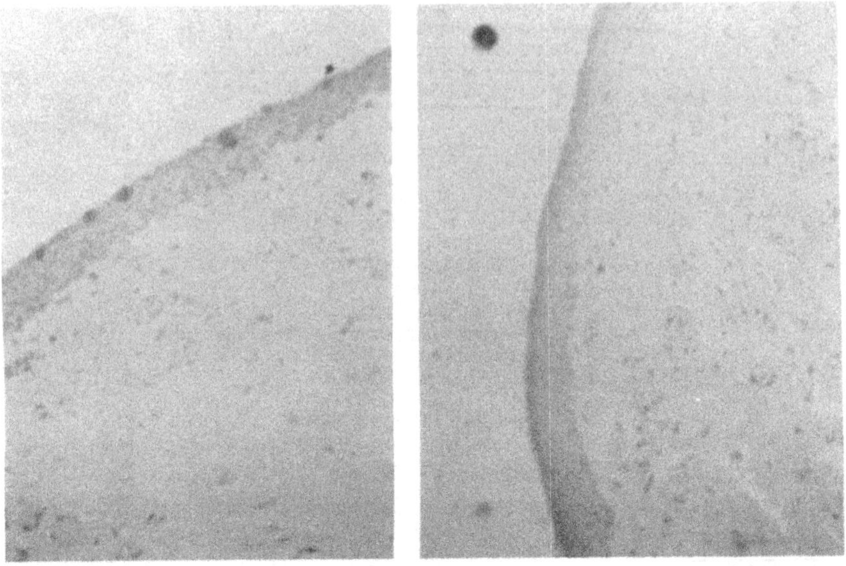

FIGURE 10: Left panel of this split-photograph shows normal human conjunctiva, with seven PAS-stained goblet cells in superficial epithelium. Right panel shows conjunctiva from a patient with CP; no goblet cells were detectable in this specimen (PAS-stain, x 250).

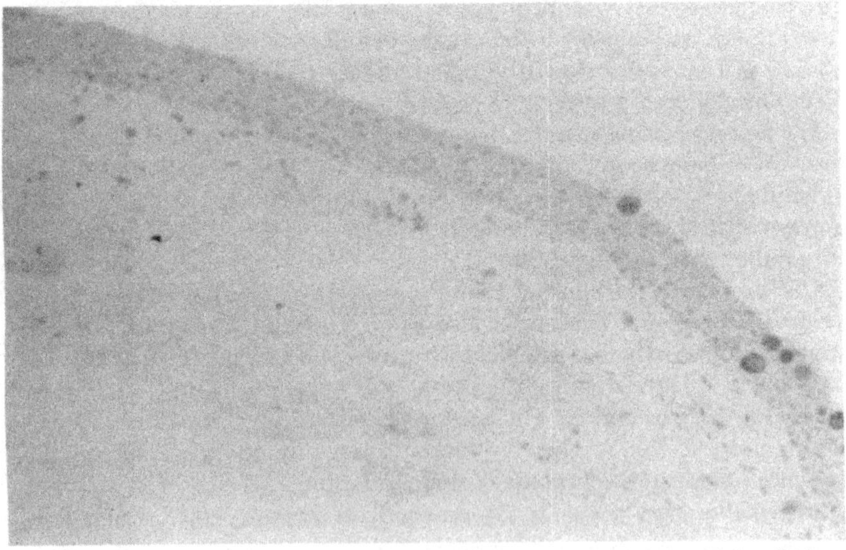

FIGURE 11: CP conjunctiva (PAS, x 100). Note presence of goblet cells in this specimen, and extreme regionality of their distribution.

TABLE X: SUMMARY OF MEAN VALUES OF CELL TYPES PER FIELD LIGHT MICROSCOPY (× 500)

	MEAN	NORMAL*	RANGE
Epithelial goblet cells	1.2	3.5	0-5
Substantia propria			
Plasma cells	29.3	4.9	5-62
Lymphocytes	24.8	4.6	3-47
Histiocytes	16.2	2.8	3-34
Mast cells	8.4	3.6	3-17
Eosinophils	1.3	1.1	0-6
Neutrophils	1.1	0	0-8

*Normal mean values reported here are taken from our analysis of 30 normal conjunctival specimens harvested at the time of cataract surgery.

Our previously unreported use of special stains, such as alkaline Giemsa, to better reveal mast cells also proved useful. The results demonstrated quite clearly that substantial mast cell participation in the substantia propria inflammatory cell infiltrate was a typical feature in all of our cases (Fig 15a, b, and c). The mast cells, scattered throughout the substantia propria, frequently were found in large numbers around venules, and often were in the process of degranulation.

In collaboration with Dr Greenwood, at Fisons, LTD, Loughboro, England, we have begun preliminary studies of the relative proportions of mast cell types in the infiltrates in CP conjunctiva. Briefly, fresh conjunctival biopsy specimens from CP patients are incubated with antibodies specific for mucosal mast cells and for connective tissue mast cells. Subsequent IF microscopy is performed to determine the presence of each type of mast cell. Normal conjunctival tissue contains small numbers of mucosal mast cells by this technique.

The preliminary results of this work confirms that mast cell numbers are increased in conjunctiva from CP patients and shows, surprisingly, that substantial numbers of connective tissue mast cells are present. Our work on this project continues, with special interest in signals responsible for mast cell recruitment and the effect of mast cell mediators on conjunctival epithelium.

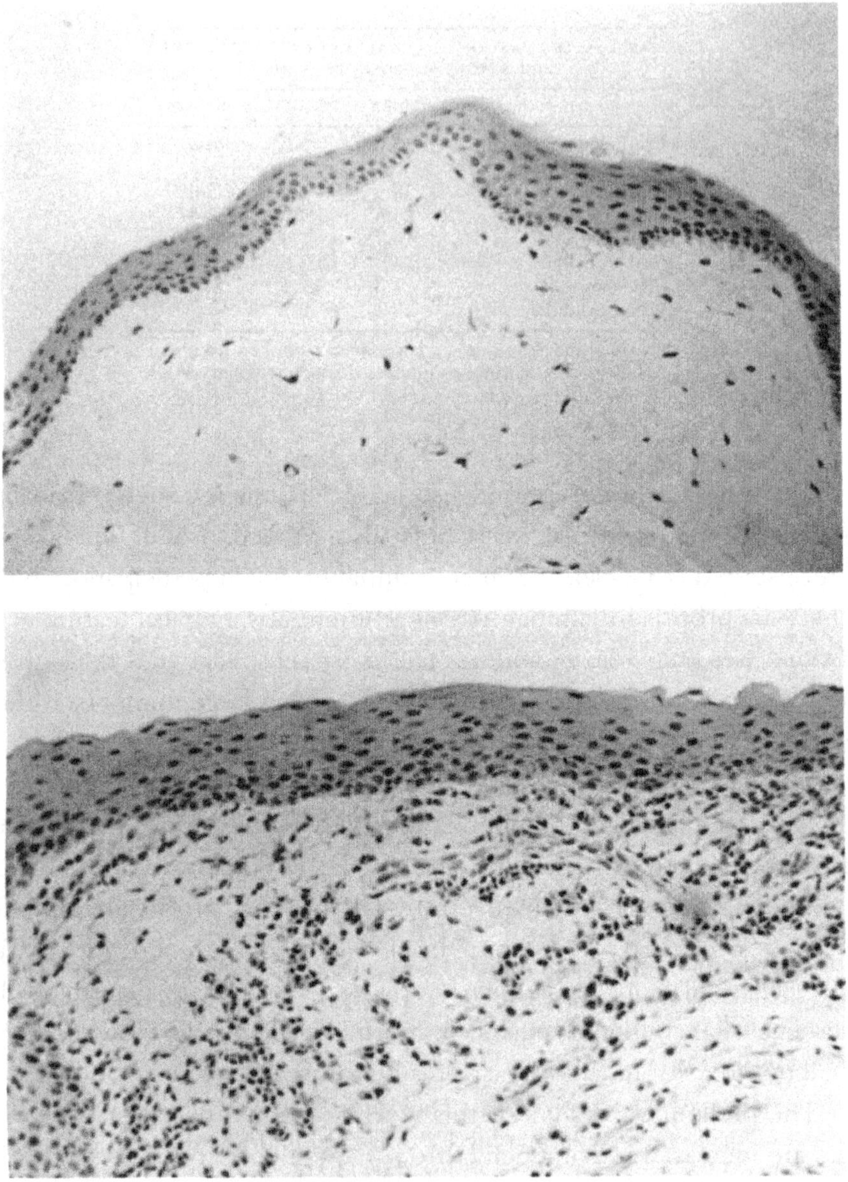

FIGURE 12: a: Normal human conjunctiva (H&E, x 200). Note, in particular, small number of mononuclear cells in substantia propria, and lack of clustering of cells around vessels. b: CP conjunctiva (H&E, x 400). In addition to squamous metaplasia of epithelium, note extreme degree of mononuclear cell infiltration of substantia propria.

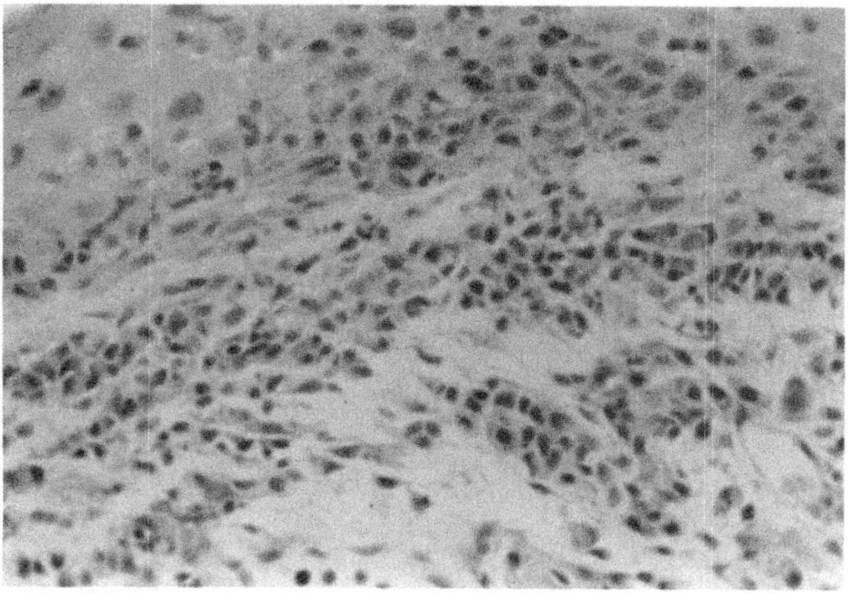

FIGURE 13: CP conjunctiva (H&E, x 160). Note extreme degree of mononuclear cell infiltration into substantia propria of conjunctiva, reaching, in some regions, almost a granulomatous appearance.

Ultrastructural Characteristics—The ultrastructural characteristics of conjunctiva affected by idiopathic CP were studied in collaboration with Dr Edward Galbavy during his fellowship at our institution. Carroll and Kuwabara[47] had reported findings on the ultrastructure of conjunctiva from one patient with pemphigoid affecting the conjunctiva. We studied three patients, comparing findings from three sites in each eye: bulbar, tarsal, and fornix conjunctiva, before and after control of the conjunctival inflammation with systemic immunosuppressive therapy. Our report has been accepted for publication.

Under local anesthesia, pretreatment biopsy specimens were taken from the conjunctiva of three patients with clinically active stage III CP. Three specimens were taken from each patient: from the inferior fornix, the lower tarsal, and the limbal area. Additional biopsy specimens were taken from two of the same patients 6 months after successful treatment with cyclophosphamide and prednisone. For comparison, biopsy specimens were also taken from conjunctiva of two normal subjects.

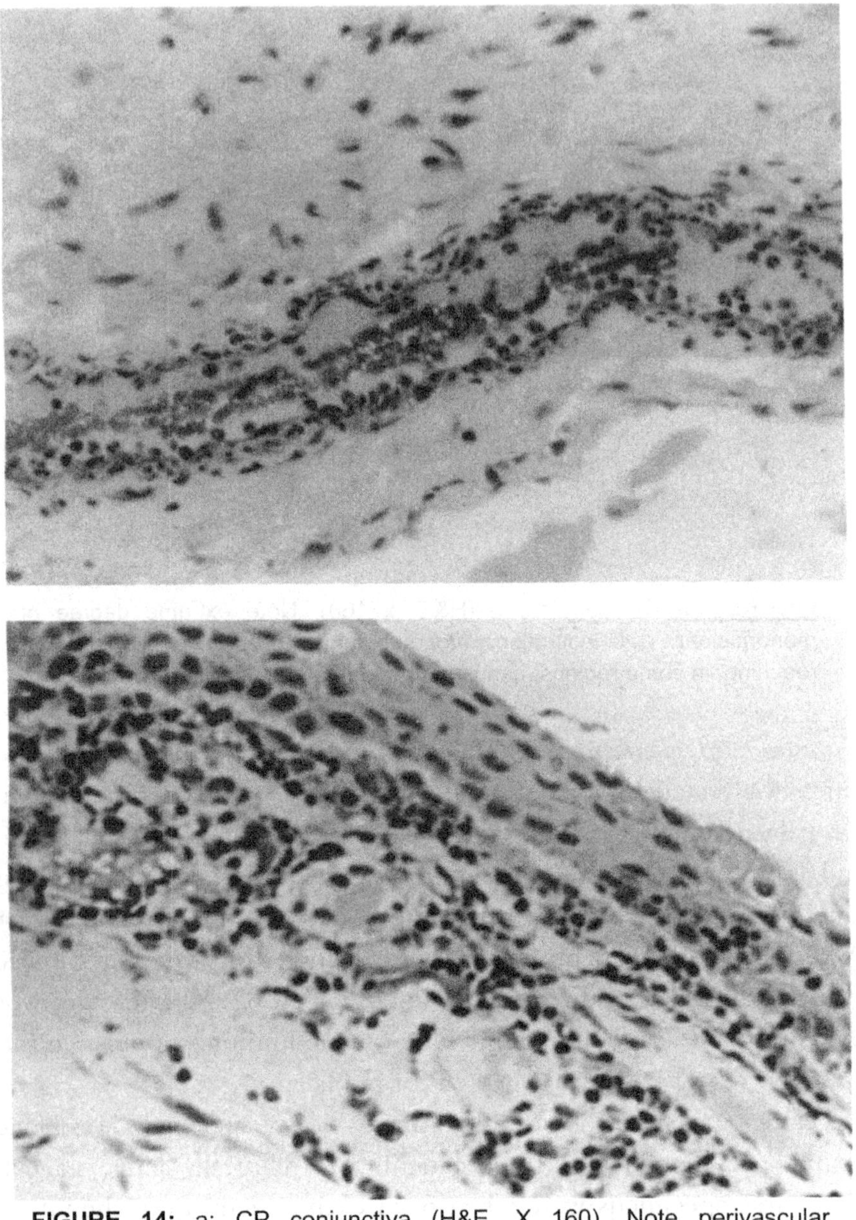

FIGURE 14: a: CP conjunctiva (H&E, X 160). Note perivascular lymphocytic "cuffing" around vessels in substantia propria in this specimen. b: CP conjunctiva (H&E, x 160). This specimen demonstrates perivascular lymphocytic infiltration.

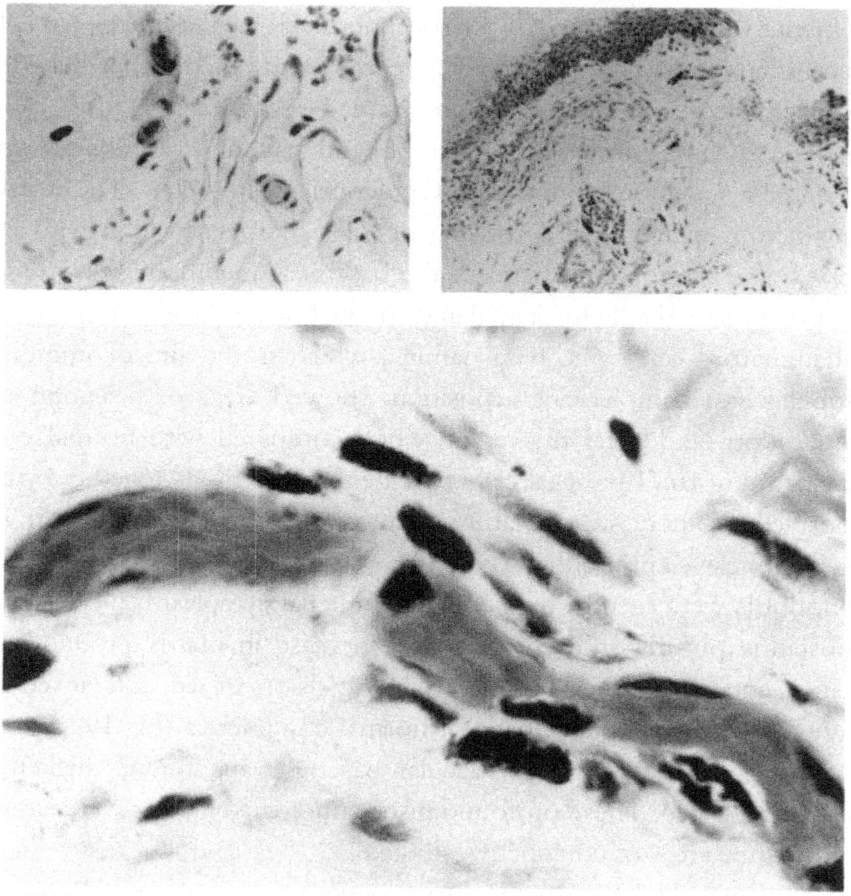

FIGURE 15: a: Normal human conjunctiva (Giemsa, X 400). One mast cell is seen directly beneath epithelium. b: CP conjunctiva (Giemsa, X 400). Eight mast cells are seen clustered around vessels in substantia propria; five mast cells in various stages of degranulation are seen in this field also. c: CP conjunctiva (Giemsa, X 1000). Extreme degrees of perivascular association of mast cells in CP conjunctival specimens was a notable characteristic finding in our studies.

Tissue specimens for transmission electron microscopy were immediately fixed in a modified Karnovsky's fixative, postfixed in osmium tetroxide, and dehydrated in ascending grades of alcohol. The specimens were then passed through propylene oxide and embedded in epon blocks. All specimens were handled identically.

An LKB ultramicrotome was used to cut thin sections, which were stained with uranyl acetate and lead citrate. A Philips 200 transmission electron microscope was used to study and photograph the conjunctival ultrastructure of the specimens. Tissue specimens for light microscopy were placed in historesin embedding media after dehydration with alcohol and processed and stained routinely.

The surface epithelium of pemphigoid patients was thinned and assumed a squamous appearance. Goblet cells were sparse. The surface cell membrane retained surprising degrees of specialization with microvilli and microplicae. Beneath the basement membrane, the lamina propria was markedly thickened and showed pronounced infiltration of inflammatory cells. The basal lamina, which is the site of immunoglobulin and complement deposition, showed areas of discontinuity, duplication, and focal thickening when compared with normal conjunctiva (Fig 16). Epithelial cells were held more closely together by the conspicuous increase of mature desmosomes, which are known for their cohesive properties (Fig 11). Prominent tonofilaments and tonofibrils were seen throughout the epithelial cytoplasm (Fig 18). The substantia propria showed a marked increase in matrix ground substance, and the collagen fibrils were highly disorganized, and lacked the bundles of fibrils characteristic of normal conjunctiva (Fig 19). Vascular space was reduced, and vascular basement membrane thickening was often noted. These profound histopathologic changes were similar in the three areas of conjunctiva studied.

Specimens of conjunctiva from patients with ocular CP treated with immunosuppressive agents were remarkable for a relative absence of desmosomes between the epithelial cells (Fig 20). Tonofibrils were likewise less prominent, and occasional goblet cells were seen. Microvilli were well-developed on the cell surface of CP patients who had been immunosuppressed.

These observations support earlier reported findings and emphasize important structural changes that are found in the conjunctiva of patients with ocular CP. In addition to the immunologic abnormalities and structural changes in the BMZ, the epithelial cells above and the lamina propria below were markedly abnormal. The squamous appearance of the epithelial cell surface is characteristic of CP at this stage. Surface specialization features of the plasma membrane (microvilli) are reduced. The enhanced network of desmosome-tonofilament complexes binds the epithelial cells tightly, providing a distinct and perhaps important clue to the pathophysiology of conjunctival surface changes. In normal skin, tonofilaments are assembled in such a way as to form many three-dimensional bundles that, when fastened to desmosomes, provide the epidermis with tonus and resist shearing stresses.[82] Some studies have attributed a limited elastic potential to tonofilaments.[83] Perhaps the surface shrinkage, fornix shortening, and symblepharon formation in CP are in part a result of the abnormalities we noted.

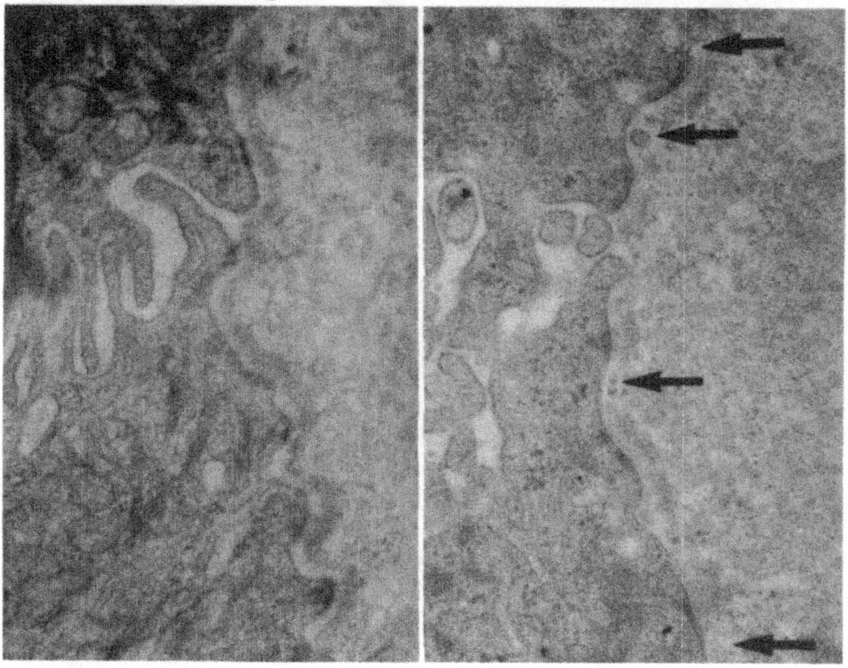

FIGURE 16: Transmission electron microscopy (X 53,900). Normal human conjunctiva is seen on left side of this split photograph. Lamina lucida and lamina densa of epithelial BMZ can be easily distinguished, with no evidence of discontinuities. Specimen on right, from a patient with CP, shows multiple areas of BMZ discontinuity (arrows).

The basal lamina of the conjunctival epithelium in CP patients was thickened and duplicated in many areas, perhaps reflecting the influence of chemical mediators (adrenergic and prostaglandin) on basement membrane production shown elsewhere in cultured corneal epithelium.[84]

The lamina propria was thickened and infiltrated by inflammatory cells. The "subepithelial fibrosis" seen on slit-lamp examination could be correlated with collagen fibrils observed among the abnormally abundant matrix material. The collagen fibrils in ocular CP appeared quite disorganized compared with the more regular arrangement in normal conjunctiva. This study did not allow us to quantify collagen deposition.

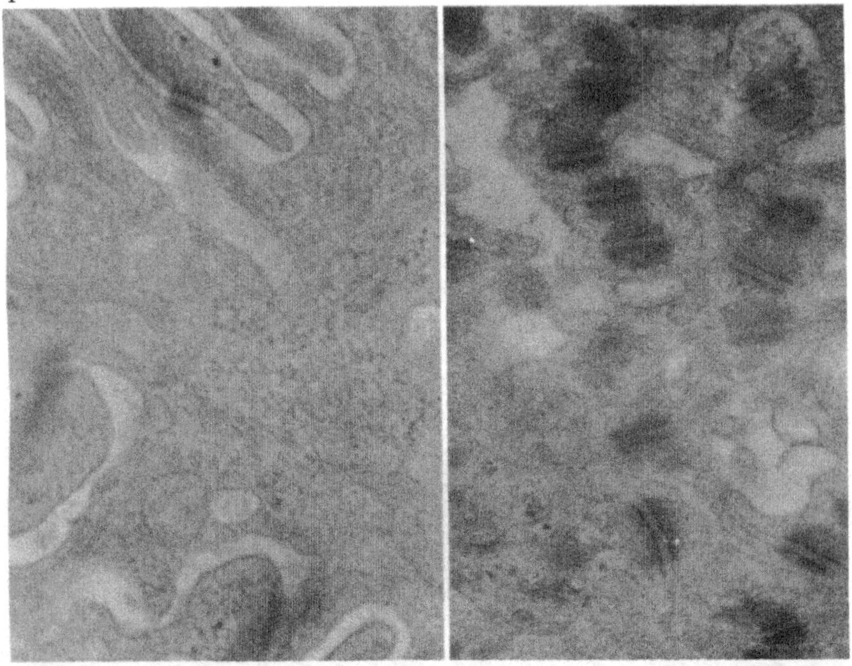

FIGURE 17: Transmission electron microscopy (x 31,000). Normal conjunctiva on left, compared with CP conjunctiva on right shows a striking difference in numbers of desmosomes anchoring adjacent epithelial cells.

Of particular interest in our postimmunosuppressive treatment specimens is the marked decrease in desmosomes and tonofibrils. The specimens were taken from patients who had dramatically improved clinically after treatment; the ultrastructural changes can thus be correlated with the clinical improvement. As we continue to observe these changes, they may prove to be important in aiding judgment of the effectiveness and dosage requirements of cytotoxic therapeutic agents. Future studies will also attempt to characterize more clearly the degree of ultrastructural alteration seen during the different stages of this disease.

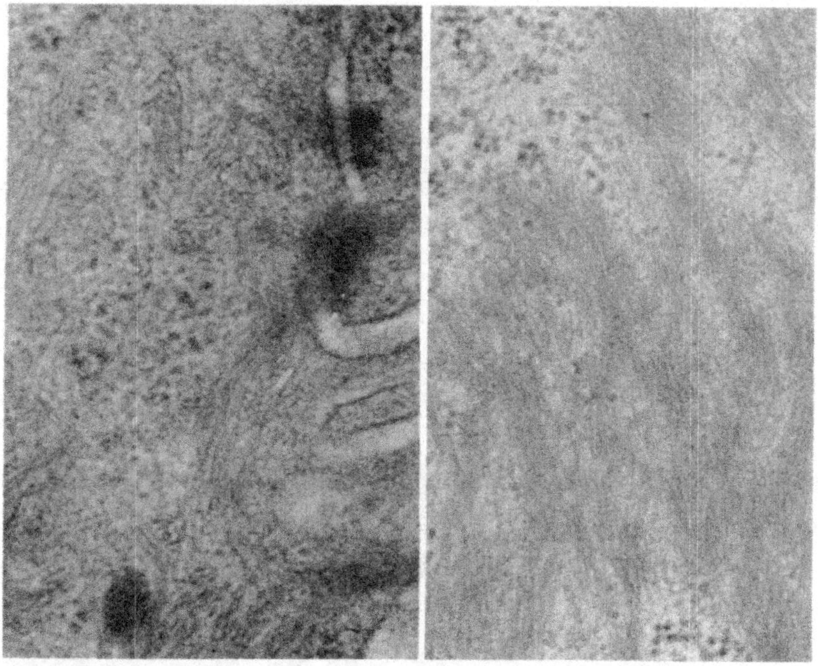

FIGURE 18: Transmission electron microscopy (x 25,900). Amount of tonofibril /tonofilament material is seen to be markedly increased in CP conjunctiva (right panel) compared to normal conjunctiva (left panel)

Drug-Induced "Pseudopemphigoid:" Light and Electron Microscopic Features— An entity known as "pseudopemphigoid" or drug-induced ocular CP has been described in association with ocular drug use.[85-89] These cases, which clinically appear indistinguishable from unilateral idiopathic pemphigoid affecting the conjunctiva, have been related to the use of echothiophate iodide,[85] pilocarpine,[86] idoxyurodine,[87] and epinephrine.[88] Interestingly, systemic practolol[89] has also been associated with bilateral conjunctival CP development. This iatrogenic form of CP, or drug-induced pseudo–pemphigoid, has never been studied by electron microscopy.

In collaboration with Professor Yves Pouliquen, Hotel-Dieu, Paris, we studied the histopathologic and ultrastructural characteristics of 22 biopsy specimens from 10 patients with iatrogenic CP affecting the conjunctiva following the use of various ocular drugs. The results of this study were reported to the American Academy of Ophthalmology, and a manuscript based on this work has been submitted for publication.

All the patients in this study presented with clinically obvious active CP affecting the conjunctiva. The eyedrops which had been used were echothiophate iodide, timolol maleate, pilocarpine, epinephrine, and dipivefrin hydrochloride. The use of all ocular medication, with the exception of lubricants, had ceased a minimum of 4 months prior to conjunctival biopsy. Cryoablation of trichitic lashes had successfully eliminated trichiasis in the four patients with trichiasis 3 months prior to biopsy. Lagophthalmus was not present in any of the patients, and all 10 patients had corneal sensations within the normal range. Patients with Stevens-Johnson syndrome, burns, sarcoidosis, atopy, trachoma, rosacea, trauma, or other possible causes of conjunctival scarring were excluded from this study. Patients with extraocular mucous membrane involvement suggestive of extraocular CP (skin, mouth, vagina) were also excluded.

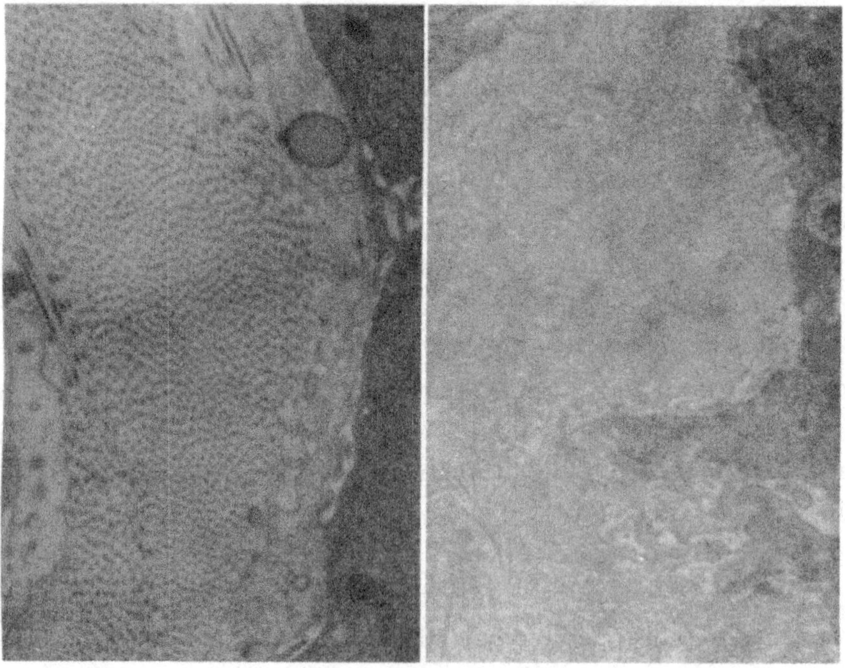

FIGURE 19: Transmission electron microscopy (X 59,300). Normal conjunctiva substantia propria, left panel, with regularly-ordered collagen bundles, compared to CP conjunctiva, right panel, with collagen fiber disorganization and increased ground matrix material.

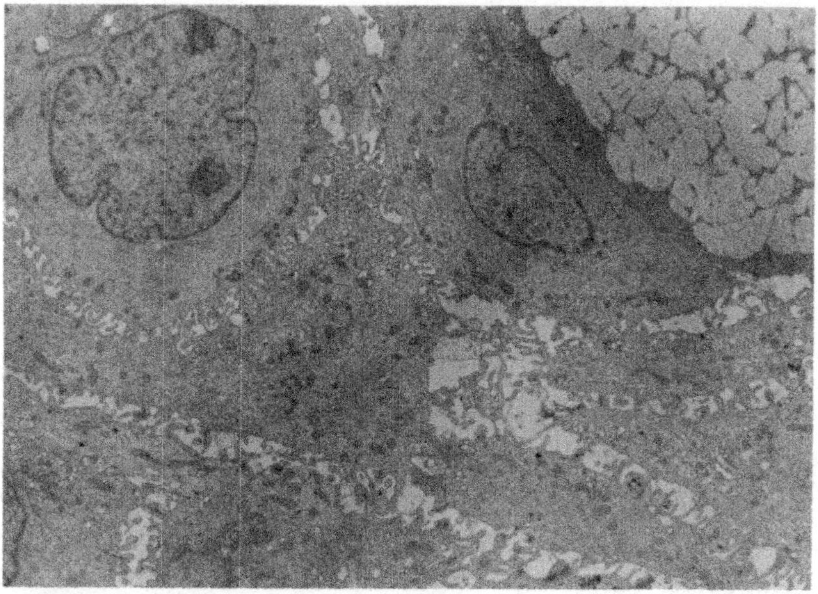

FIGURE 20: Transmission electron microscopy (x 7200). Conjunctival specimen from successfully treated (immunosuppressed) CP patient. Note resultant reversal of intense desmosome and tonofibril system seen in untreated patient specimens.

Biopsy specimens were taken by me from bulbar conjunctiva, the fornix, and inferior tarsal conjunctiva; the ultrastructural study was performed in Dr Pouliquen's laboratory.

There were 22 biopsies from 10 patients (3 men and 7 women) all at stage III of the disease. Demographic data concerning the age, sex, and the drug used are reported in Table XI.

Six patients had biopsy specimens taken from all three conjunctival sites. Two patients had only one biopsy from the limbus and two others only from the fornix. The tissue specimens were fixed in 2.5% glutaraldehyde in phosphate-buffered saline (PBS), pH 7.2, with postfixation in 2% osmium in cacodylate buffer. They were then stained with 4% uranyl acetate and 0.4% lead citrate in 0.1 N sodium hydroxide, dehydrated in acetone and propylene oxide, and embedded in epon. This sections for transmission electron microscopy were analyzed with a Philips 300 transmission electron microscope at 60 V accelerating voltage.

TABLE XI

CASE	AGE/SEX	DRUG
1	82 F	Pilocarpine
2	53 M	Timolol
3	67 F	Pilocarpine
4	62 F	Pilocarpine
5	68 F	Epinephrine
6	78 M	Epinephrine
7	68 F	Phosphate iodine
8	72 F	Phosphate iodine
9	90 F	Pilocarpine Epinephrine
10	60 M	Timolol

One-micron sections for light microscopy were stained with toluidine blue.

The goblet cell density was measured and graded as + + when normal, + when diminished, and 0 when the specimen was devoid of goblet cells. The normal density, in our experience, is 11 cells/mm^2. Epithelial thickness was correlated with the number of cellular layers and was graded + when the epithelium showed more than five layers and - when less than five. Keratinization was graded + when abnormal superficial keratinization was visible and - when not. This judgment was based on morphology typical of squamous metaplasia.

Substantia propria vascularization was arbitrarily graded using a reference field of 0.02 mm^2; a grade of + + + designated vascularized areas larger than 50%, + + designated 25% to 50%, + from 5% to 25%, and - when less than 5%. This analysis was performed twice on each specimen at two different subepithelial depths: one immediately under the basal membrane, and the other deeper in the substantia propria. Normal bulbar, tarsal, and fornix conjunctiva was similarly studied as a control.

Inflammatory cell types were counted collectively. Inflammation was graded + + + when more than 50 inflammatory cells were found per field, + + for 25 to 50 cells, + for 5 to 25 cells, and - when fewer than 5 were seen. All the results are shown in Table XII.

All parameters studied by light microscopy were reexamined and confirmed by electron microscopy. But with this technique precise quantification of each parameter is not possible, and therefore the electron microscope observations are classically descriptive.

Goblet cells were absent in 14 of the 22 biopsy specimens. In two patients this absence was found on three sites of biopsy. Goblet cells were decreased in six biopsies, three of which were from one patient. Goblet cell numbers were normal in three biopsy specimens from two patients.

TABLE XII*

CASE	BIOPSY SITE	GOBLET CELLS	EPITHELIAL CHANGES	INFLAMMATION	VASCULARIZATION	
					SS	DEEP
1	L	0	K/S	+ + +	−	+ + +
	T	0	K/S	+ + +	−	−
	F	0	K/S	+ + +	−	−
2	L	0	K/S	+ +	−	+
	T	+ +	None	+	+	+
	F	+ +	None	+ +	+ +	+ +
3	L	+	None	+	+	+ +
	T	+	None	+	−	+ + +
	F	+	None	+ +	−	+
4	L	0	K/S	+	+ +	+ + +
	T	0	K/S	−	+	+ +
	F	0	K/S	−	+ + +	+ + +
5	L	+	K	+ + +	−	−
	T	0	S	+ + +	−	+
	F	0	K/S	+ + +	+	+
6	L	0	K/S	+	+	+ +
	T	0	K/S	+	+	+
	F	+	None	+	+	+ +
7	L	0	K/S	+	+	+
8	L	+ +	None	−	+ +	+ + +
9	F	0	S	+ + +	−	+ + +
10		0	Very thin	+ + +	−	−

*SS = superficial stroma, L = limbal, T = tarsal, F = fornix, K = keratinization, S = stratification.

The absence of goblet cells did not seem correlated to the site of biopsy; three normal goblet cell densities were found; one in the limbal, one in the tarsal, and one in the fornix zone.

In 11 specimens the epithelium was superficially keratinized, with abnormally increased stratification. Two patients showed squamous metaplasia at all three sites of biopsy. In one specimen superficial keratinization was apparent and hyperstratification was observed in two others. In seven specimens, three of which were from the same patient, the epithelium appeared normal. One specimen from a patient biopsied only at one site was not interpretable due to an extreme thinning of the epithelium.

In eight biopsy specimens the inflammatory cell density of subjacent connective tissue was higher than 50 cells/0.02 mm^2 Two of these specimens were from two patients; and six were from two other patients. Three specimens from two patients had a density of 25 to 50 cells; eight specimens from five patients had a density of 5 to 25 cells; and three specimens from two patients had fewer than 5 cells.

Normal reference conjunctiva consistently showed a loose connective tissue with an average vascular space of slightly greater than 50% of the 0.02 mm^2 reference field.

In biopsy specimens from six patients the vascular space was less than 5% of the surface analyzed. One patient showed this feature at all three biopsy sites. In eight specimens (biopsies from six patients) the vascular space was 5% to 25%. The vascular space was 25% to 50% in three specimens from three patients, and was more than 50% in one specimen. This specimen was taken from the fornix of a patient who was also biopsied in tarsal and bulbar conjunctiva; these two other sites showed different degrees of vascularization (25% to 50% at the limbus and 5% to 25% in the tarsal specimen).

The percentage value of vascularized area could not be correlated with any particular site of biopsy. All the values noted above have been observed immediately under the basal lamina. In the deeper region of the substantia propria we observed that the vascular space was equal to (10 specimens) or greater than (12 specimens) the value for the same section immediately subepithelial.

Electron Microscopy of Superficial Epithelial Cells. The superficial epithelial cells appeared flattened. Their cytoplasm showed an abnormal density of tonofibrils. Large vacuoles filled with granular amorphous material and a high concentration of glycogen particles were also observed in the cytoplasm of these cells. The nuclei were absent. Intercellular spaces were rare in the superficial area, and those that persisted were filled with a granular material. Cell-to-cell junctions in the superficial area consisted of large numbers of deep interdigitations with increased numbers of desmosomes (Fig 21).

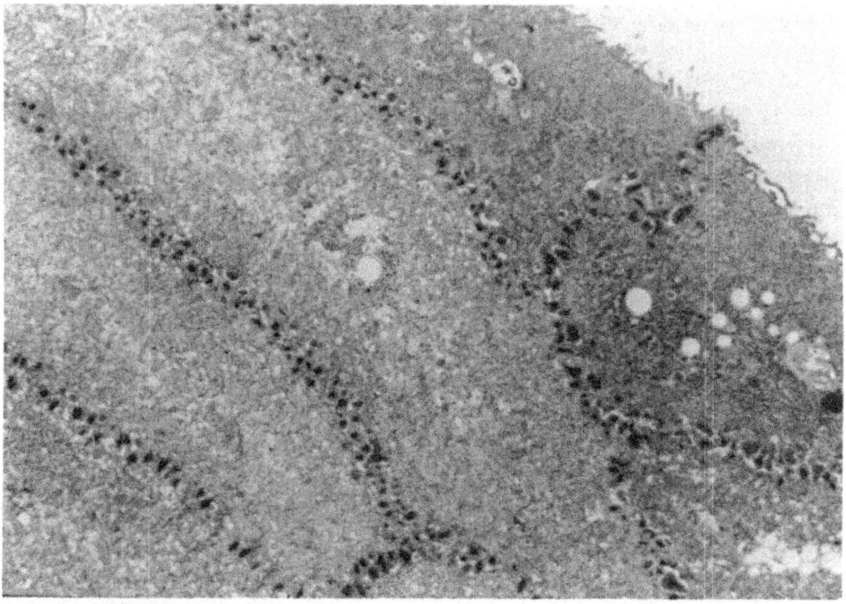

FIGURE 21: Transmission electron microscopy (X 8500). "Pseudopemphigoid" conjunctival epithelium. Just as in idiopathic CP, epithelium has lost its normal loose connections, and cells are tightly joined with numerous desmosomes (d). Vacuoles (v) are abundant in cytoplasm with accumulation of glycogen and increased tonofibrils.

Goblet cells, though rare, appeared ultrastructurally normal, with rich, rough-surfaced endoplasmic reticulum and mitochondria, and varying amounts of granules.

Basal cells showed an abnormal number of tonofibrils often packed together in large bundles linked to desmosomes (Fig 22). Signs of increased intracellular activity were present (ie, hyperdeveloped Golgi and endoplasmic reticulum).

Numerous pinocytotic vesicles were located at the basal pole of these cells. Intercellular spaces were present between the cells and their occasional dilation suggested the existence of epithelial edema. They were often filled with a granular material or with inflammatory cells.

The basal lamina features were heterogeneous. The basal lamina was continuous in only 4 of 22 specimens. Derangements included breaks and discontinuity (in 10 of 22 specimens), but without any duplication. Eight of the 22 specimens showed reduplication of three or four irregular and thickened layers (Fig 23).

Some portions of the basal lamina remained attached to the basal cells by a few hemidesmosomes, but most often there were no attachments between the basal epithelial layer and the underlying basal lamina. In such cases, we often observed "basal lamina-like" structures in the adjacent connective tissue.

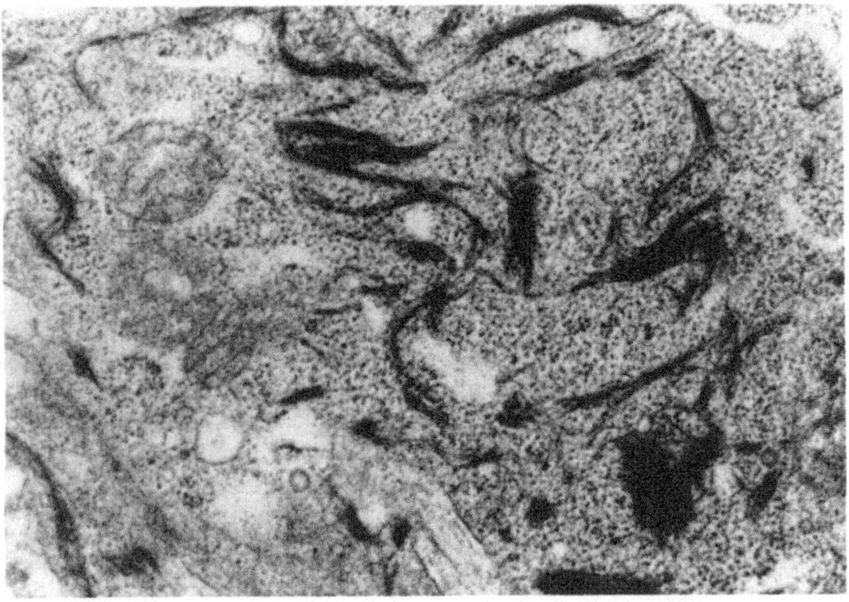

FIGURE 22: Transmission electron microscopy (x 7050). Cytoplasm of all epithelial cells, including basal cells, shown here, arranged in large bundles.

Substantia Propria. The substantia propria was thicker, and richer in fibrous material, in collagen and elastin, and in necrotic cellular debris than was normal human conjunctiva (or normal substantia propria).

The collagen fibril arrangement was modified in the substantia propria of patients with drug-induced CP. New collagen formation was obvious; these fibers were more compact and were organized in large bundles, with an apparent diminution of the interfibrillar space. They often appeared with radiating bundles in "flower petal" pattern (Fig 24).

Fiber diameter was heterogeneous, and fibers varied from simple to double. The nature of the granular amorphous material frequently observed between the fibers is unknown.

This connective tissue was also rich in elastic fibers visualized in two forms. One, amorphous and electron-dense, was interpreted to be elastin, while the other component was microfibrillar. The microfibrillar material was always located near the amorphous component and stained strongly with lead citrate or uranyl acetate.

Lymphatic and blood vessels reflected the inflammatory process by the presence of numerous microvesicles in the endothelial cell cytoplasm. Sometimes large vesicles were visible (probably resulting from coalescence of smaller ones). Cell membranes appeared quite irregular where these large vesicles opened to the extracellular space.

The vascular features varied from an endothelial cell hypertrophy, with possible closure of the intravascular lumen, to endothelial cell death, discernible by the vacuolization of the cytoplasm, presence of pyknotic nucleus and disappearance of the cell membrane.

The vascular basal lamina was often thicker, and duplication was observed in some sections (Fig 25).

The cellular population was typically composed of active fibroblasts, lymphocytes, plasma cells and mast cells in 16 of 22 specimens. Fibroblasts exhibited well-developed intracytoplasmic cell constituents, including Golgi apparatus and granular endoplasmic reticulum whose dilated cisternae often contained fine granular material. The increased cellular activity was also evident from the presence of numerous vesicles arranged along the cell membranes.

The mast cells were observed principally in superficial perivenular locations.

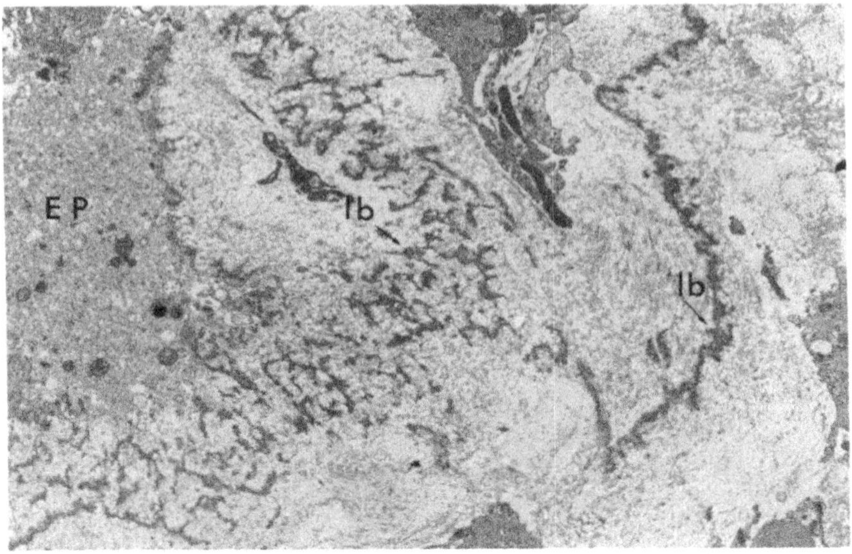

FIGURE 23: Transmission electron microscopy (X 22,300). Massive reduplication of basal lamina material in "pseudopemphigoid" conjunctiva specimen. Basal lamina (BL) is seen irregularly arranged under basal epithelium (EP).

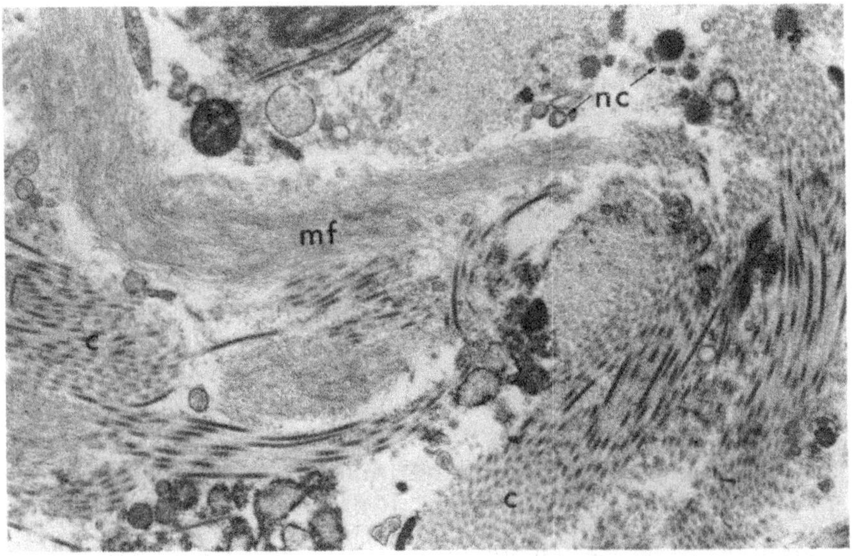

FIGURE 24: Transmission electron microscopy (X 17,800). Irregularly arranged collagen bundles (C), elastin microfibrils (mF), and areas of collagen necrosis (CN).

The plasma cells, lymphocytes, or activated lymphocytes with prominent nucleoli inside an enlarged nucleus and with chromatin arranged along the nuclear membrane, appeared scattered in the connective tissue, and their density seemed well correlated with vascular damage (Fig 26).

Neutrophils were found in only three sites from two subjects. No appreciable number of eosinophils was noted.

Despite the identical clinical status of all the patients, the features seen by light and electron microscopy were varied, not only from patient to patient, but also from one biopsy site to the other in the same patient. None of the medications could be associated with specific changes. Nor was there any preferential site of involvement in the conjunctiva, as all areas of the conjunctiva can be involved at various stages independently in CP.

In these cases, the number of conjunctival goblet cells was lower than in normal conjunctiva. In about half of our cases they were totally absent.

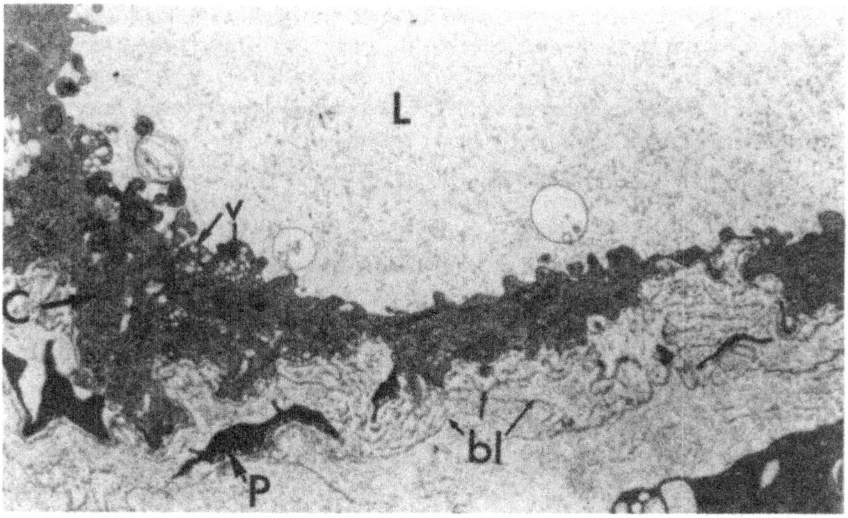

FIGURE 25: Transmission electron microscopy (X 17,800). Vasculopathy with a routine finding in "pseudopemphigoid" conjunctival specimens. Here endothelial cell (EC) is highly vacuolated (v) (evidence of a high degree of metabolic activity), and has manufactured large amounts of basal lamina material (bL).

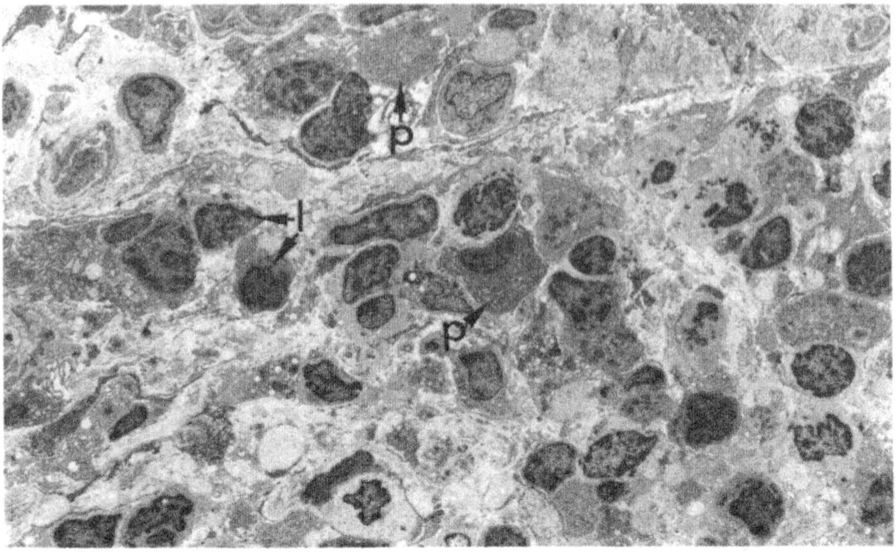

FIGURE 26: Plasma cells (p) and lymphocytes (l) are metabolically highly active, with large amounts of mitochondria and endoplasmic reticulum (X 2200).

In the biopsies studied, the absence of goblet cells was associated with an intense underlying inflammation (more than 25 cells/0.02 mm^2 in 8 of 14 cases) and with a decrease in vascularity (0.25%/0.02 mm^2).

These observations are similar to those of Tseng and associates[42] who found a loss of goblet cells in conjunctival biopsy specimens of diverse pathologies associated with minimum vascularization or intense inflammation.

Carroll and Kuwabara[47] noted on electron microscopy the absence of goblet cells in the bulbar conjunctival biopsies of one patient with idiopathic CP. It seems important to emphasize that we found an occasional goblet cell in an advanced stage (stage III) of conjunctival cicatrization in three biopsies. The presence of these cells in iatrogenic, drug-induced ocular CP contrasts with the reports of Hirst et al[86] and Patten et al.[85]

In our cases where the goblet cells were either markedly diminished or absent, we observed marked alteration of the epithelium (an increase in stratification and keratinization). These alterations are never found when goblet cells are abundant.

This finding leads us to hypothesize that the disappearance of goblet cells is an early sign of epithelial transdifferentiation; reduced vascularization may have at least a partial effect on the epithelium. Additional preliminary experiments in our laboratories suggest that inflammatory events in the substantia propria may play a profound role in the status of the ocular surface epithelium.

Although the studies of Carroll and Kuwabara[47] were performed on idiopathic CP, it should be noted that their observations are identical to ours except for the occasional presence of goblet cells in our specimens.

We noted, on electron microscopy, advanced parakeratinization associated with flattening of superficial and intermediate epithelial cells, intracytoplasmic keratofibrils, numerous desmosomes, and a reduction or complete disappearance of intercellular spaces. The trans-differentiation to squamous epithelium is diffuse and not restricted to areas of symblepharon.

We did not find any basal lamina modification different from that already discussed by Carroll and Kuwahara.[47] Reduplication and fragmentation of the basement membrane are not specific for CP; I have observed these features in cases of allergic keratoconjunctivitis as well. Wintroub et al,[90] Andersen et al,[44] and Dvorak et al[91] found an elevated number of eosinophils in skin biopsy specimens from patients with bullous pemphigoid of the skin; we did not observe an abnormal number of these cells in our conjunctival specimens.

The response of the microvascular system to chronic inflammation has been only minimally studied ultrastructurally. One of the signs of pathologic involvement of the vascular system is the appearance of vacuoles and microvesicles in capillary endothelial cells. Carter et al[92] have proposed that the vacuoles may be associated with the ability of macromolecules to permeate capillaries.

The thickening of perivascular basal lamina and the endothelial cell alterations observed in our study are characteristic of repeated attempts at repair by the vascular endothelium. We propose, in agreement with Susi and Shklar,[93] that thickening of the epithelial basal lamina in CP may also result from reparative processes.

Given the identical histopathology, immunopathology (personal observations), and therapeutic response to immunosuppressive agents (personal observations) of drug-induced and idiopathic CP, we wonder if drug-induced pseudopemphigoid develops in individuals who are destined to develop pemphigoid and who, by chance, also have an ocular disorder requiring the use of one of the medications reported above. It is possible that such drug use stimulates more rapid emergence of the chronic cicatrizing features of CP. We would note further that we have now observed definitive CP changes in the untreated eyes of four patients with unilateral drug-induced pseudopemphigoid.

Scanning Electron Microscopy of Conjunctival Surfaces in CP Patients—We studied the ultrastructural morphology of the conjunctival surface in patients with CP and in normal individuals. This work was conducted by my laboratory technician, Ms Carolyn De Siena and Dr Peter Wells, a post-doctoral fellow.

Decreased numbers of observable conjunctival goblet cells coupled with decreased tear film stability and eventual tear insufficiency in CP patients have led some to characterize CP as a "mucin deficient dry eye syndrome."[78,80] Our patients with active, progressive CP, however, commonly complain of excess mucus production. Indeed, strands of mucus-like material are often found in the inferior fornix of these patients during slit-lamp examination.

Human ocular mucus[94] had been studied with scanning electron microscopy, but the conjunctival surface in CP has not. Although the primary focus of this study was active CP, additional patients whose disease was controlled with immunosuppressive agents were also studied to determine if any of the ultrastructural changes observed in active CP were reversible with drug therapy. We studied the conjunctival surface of patients with CP in order to: (1) characterize the surface specializations present, (2) determine whether any ocular surface abnormalities were associated with active disease, and (3) study the relationship between the surface specializations and ocular mucus.

Conjunctival biopsy specimens were harvested from ten patients with active CP, three patients whose CP was controlled with cytotoxic drug therapy, and six normal control patients undergoing cataract surgery. After subconjunctival injection of 2% xylocaine, a 2 X 2 mm^2 section of limbal conjunctiva was removed and placed immediately on a small piece of fixative-saturated cardboard. The specimen, along with the anchoring card-board was placed in Karnovsky's fixative (1% paraformaldehyde, 1.25% glutaraldehyde, 25 mmol/l sodium phosphate, and 150 mmol/l sodium cacodylate, pH 7.2) for 24 to 48 hours and then washed with 0.2 mol/l sodium cacodylate buffer. The tissue was then dehydrated with a series of graded ethanol solutions, washed three times with absolute ethanol, and critical point dried using liquid carbon dioxide. The dried specimens were attached to aluminum stubs with silver paint, sputter-coated with gold, and viewed with an AMR 1200 scanning electron microscope.

In a separate study, half of each specimen was processed routinely for scanning electron microscopy and the second half treated with 20% N-acetyl-cysteine (Mucomyst) using a technique for the removal of ocular surface mucus.[95] These specimens were first fixed with Karnovsky's fixative for 40 minutes in order to preserve the normal morphologic characteristics, and then placed in 20% N-acetyl-cysteine for 10 minutes. Fixation with Karnovsky's fixative was repeated for 10 minutes followed by a second 10-minute treatment with Mucomyst before the specimen was transferred to Karnovsky's fixative for 24 to 48 hours. The specimens were then dehydrated with graded ethanol solutions and processed as outlined above for scanning electron microscopy.

Scanning electron microscopy specimens to be prepared for transmission electron microscopy were removed from the stubs by cutting through the silver paint just below the specimen with a razor blade. The specimens were immediately transferred to 95% ethanol overnight,[96] washed with absolute ethanol followed by acetone, and embedded in epon-araldite mixture.[97] Thin sections were cut from the blocks with a diamond knife, mounted on copper mesh grids, stained with 2% aqueous uranyl acetate, and observed with a JEOL-100C transmission electron microscope.

We found normal human conjunctival surface features identical to those previously described.[94,98,99] The epithelial surface showed extensive specialization with microplicae, microvilli, and some elongated microvillus projections (Fig 27a) present. In some areas of the conjunctiva, the epithelial cell borders were demarcated by raised ridges with tufting of the microvilli in the central regions of the cells (Fig 27b).

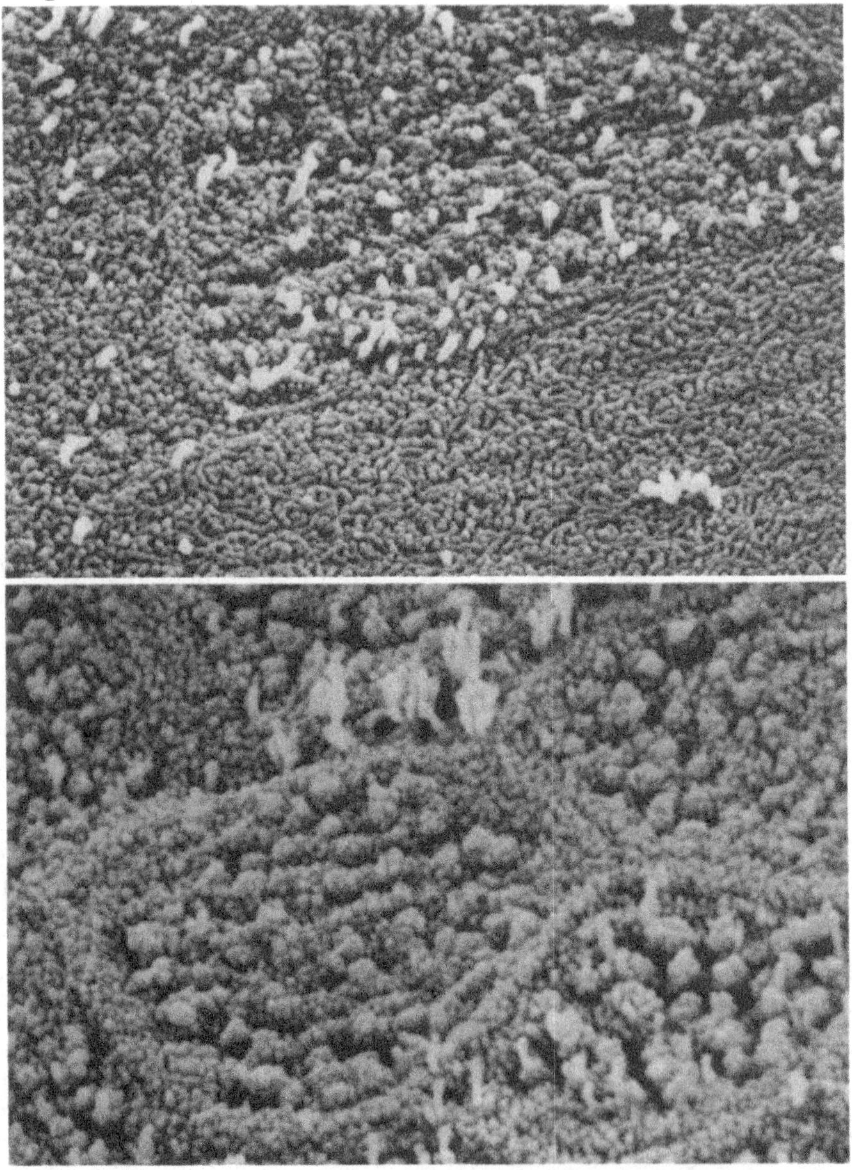

FIGURE 27: a: Scanning electron microscopy (SEM) (X 7800). Normal human conjunctiva. Note rich "carpet'" of surface specializations with microplicae, microvilli, and occasional elongated microvillus projections. b: SEM, normal human conjunctiva (x 8000). Note epithelial cell borders and occasional tufting of microvilli.

The most striking feature of the active CP conjunctival tissue was the presence of an amorphous sheet of mucus-like material covering extensive areas of the surface (Fig 28). This material often obscured the microvilli of the underlying epithelial cells and sometimes appeared granular, with knob-like bulbs extending from the surface of the sheet. At higher magnification, this sheet of material appeared closely associated with the microvilli of the cell surface (Fig 29). Ropy and twirled extensions of the sheet were noted in specimens from several patients with active CP (Fig 30). The sheet was occasionally discontinuous, allowing observation of the underlying epithelium. Mucomyst treatment of specimens from patients with active disease reduced much of the surface sheet, leaving only residual strands of mucus along the borders of the surface cells (Fig 31). The epithelium of the active CP patients closely resembled that of normal conjunctival tissue. Microplicae and microvilli were plentiful in CP patients (Fig 32). Cells with tufted microvilli and elongated microvillus projections were often observed in active CP patients, as were raised epithelial cell borders.

Correlative transmission electron microscopic observations of scanning electron microscopy specimens from patients with active CP demonstrated that the sheet of mucus-like material overlying the microvilli of the surface cells was approximately 0.12 to 0.20 μm thick (Fig 33). These transmission electron microscopic observations clearly differentiated ocular mucus from fibrin clots containing erythrocytes, which were occasionally present at the periphery of the specimen. These clots resulted from microhemorrhage of the stromal vessels at the cut edges of the biopsy. Fibrin clots were also distinguished from ocular mucus by the smaller, uniform diameter of the fibrin filaments, and the presence of erythrocytes within the clot.

The thick sheet of mucus material seen on the conjunctival surface in patients with active CP was not observed in any of the specimens from patients whose CP was drug-controlled (Fig 34). The epithelial cells were clearly visible in controlled CP, and surface specializations were evident. Microvilli, microplicae, elongated microvillus projections, and tufted microvilli were observed on the cell surfaces.

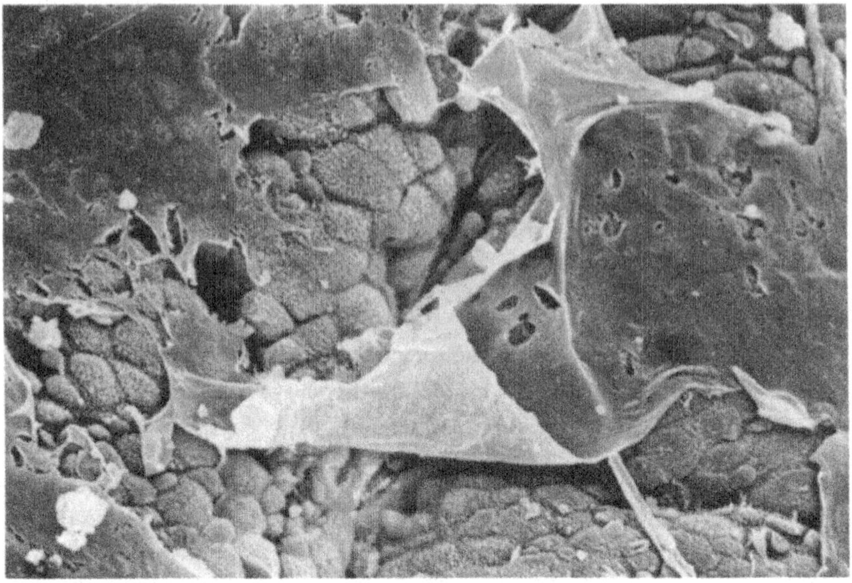

FIGURE 28: SEM, CP conjunctiva (X 1040). Note amorphous sheet of material covering most of surface of conjunctival epithelium.

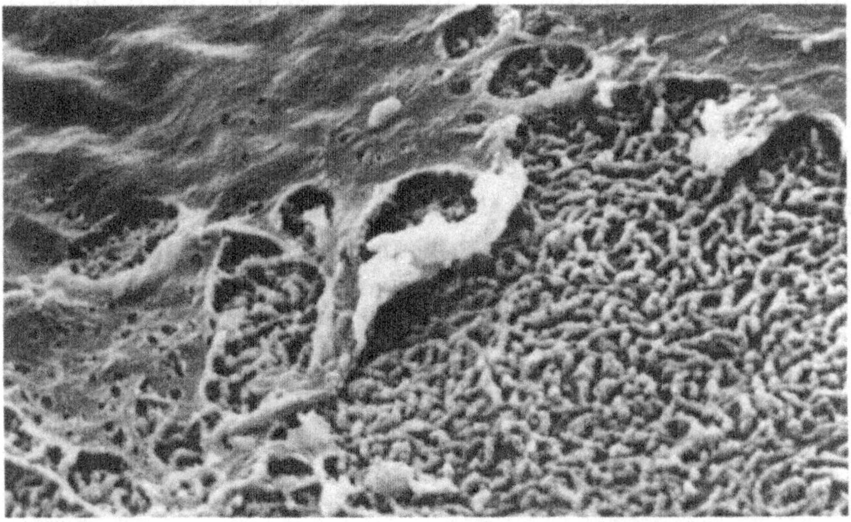

FIGURE 29: SEM, CP conjunctiva (x 9800). Amorphous sheet appears tightly attached to relatively normal appearing microvilli and microplicae underneath.

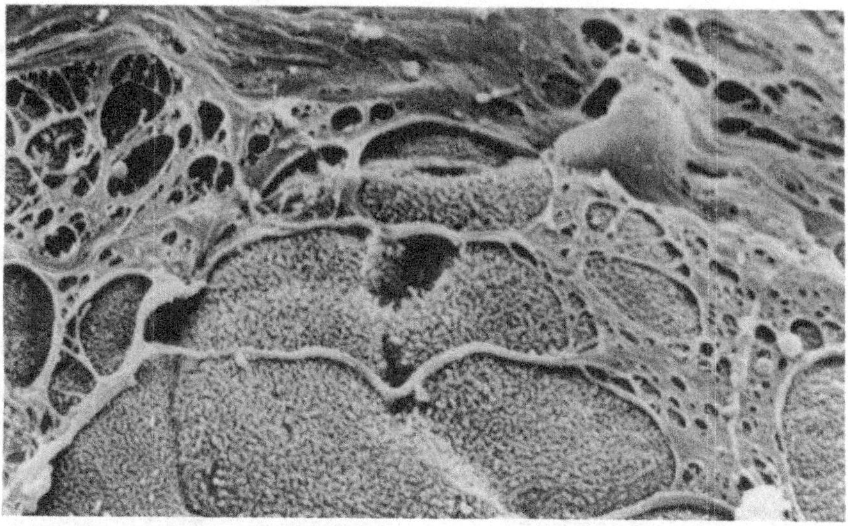

FIGURE 30: SEM, CP conjunctiva (X 3400). Discontinuous amorphous sheet with underlying rich" carpet" of surface specializations easily seen.

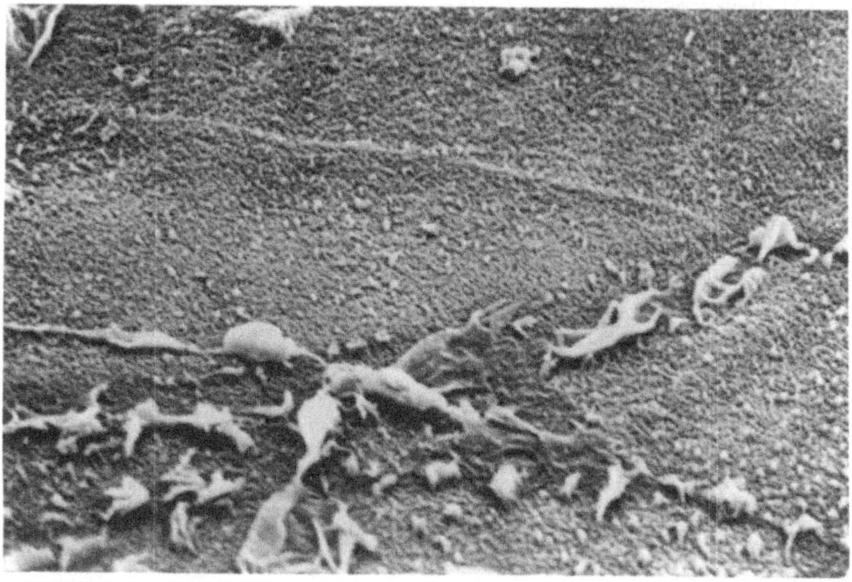

FIGURE 31: SEM, CP conjunctiva, after treatment with N-acetyl cysteine (x 3600). Only a small amount of amorphous sheet remains after pre-treatment of specimen with mucolytic agent , Mucomyst.

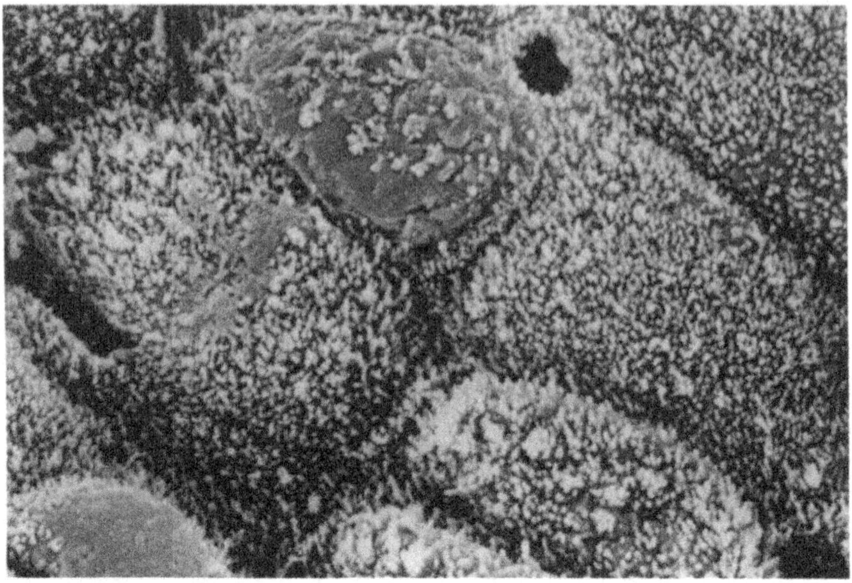

FIGURE 32: SEM, CP conjunctiva (X 3900). Specimen from CP patient showing an area with only patches of thick mucus sheet. Microvilli, microplicae, tufted microvilli, and epithelial cell borders are visible on conjunctival surface.

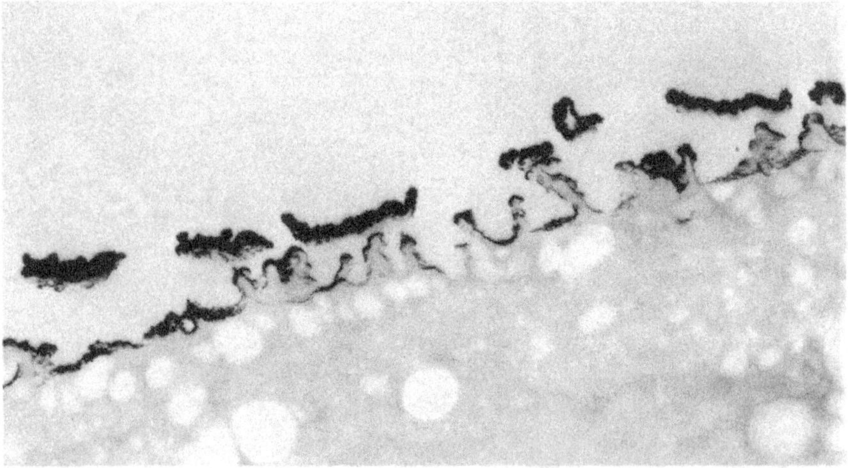

FIGURE 33: Transmission electron microscopy (TEM) of specimen previously processed for scanning electron microscopy (SEM). Specimen from patient with active CP (X 28,000). Correlative TEM of the SEM specimens confirmed presence of a sheet of material which resembles appearance of mucus on TEM.

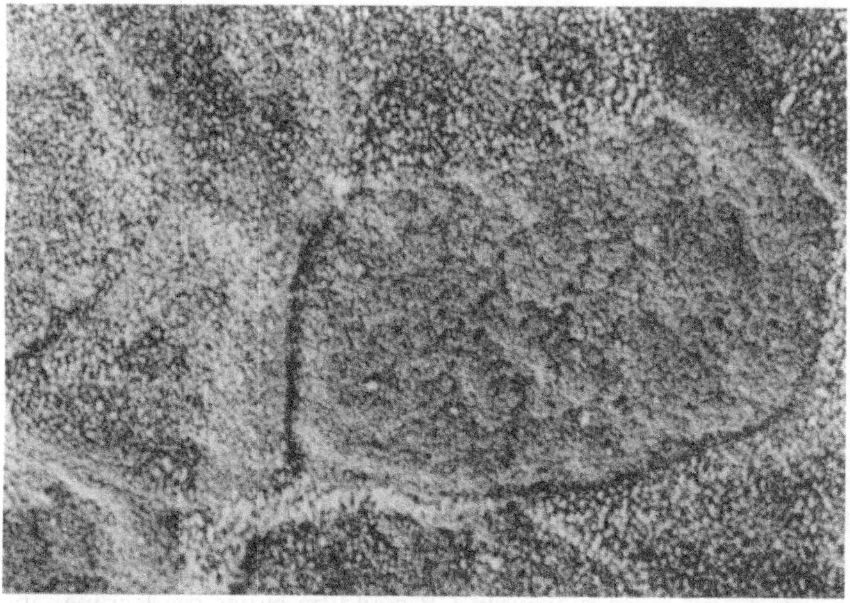

FIGURE 34: SEM (x 3600). Specimen from CP patient successfully controlled on immunosuppressive chemotherapy. Note complete absence of any amorphous sheet, and easily observable rich "carpet" of surface specializations.

Previous scanning electron microscope studies of normal human ocular mucus[94,99] have shown that it consists of strands, granules, and mucus sheets that sometimes appear as a network of mucous strands. The mucus sheet in CP generally appeared thicker and more continuous than the mucus seen on the conjunctival surface of the normal individuals in both this and previous studies.[94,99] Furthermore, our findings indicated that a thicker, more continuous sheet of mucus exists on the conjunctival surface of patients with active CP than on the conjunctiva of patients with drug-controlled CP. At this point, we can only speculate that its presence is related to the disease state. The partial degradation of this amorphous sheet with 20% N-acetyl-cysteine (Mucomyst) and our correlative transmission electron microscope observations indicate that the sheet observed in active CP consists primarily of ocular mucus. Studies of tracheo-bronchial mucus 100 have shown that the addition of deoxyribonucleic acid (DNA) or protein to mucus causes an increase in the viscosity of the mucus gel. The thick sheet of mucus material overlying the conjunctival surface in active CP could represent ocular mucus which has been contaminated with proteins and nucleic acid from desquamating or rupturing epithelial cells. Thus, the modified mucus layer may be a by-product of chronic inflammation.

Although histologic studies of patients with active CP[101-103] have shown that the density of conjunctival goblet cells is drastically reduced in this disease, several biochemical studies[102,104] have demonstrated that patients with active CP possess measurable amounts of mucin glycoprotein. Additional studies by our group (described later) using polyacrylamide gel electrophoresis have shown that patients with active CP have mucin glycoproteins that are indistinguishable from the mucin glycoproteins of normal individuals or individuals with other types of ocular inflammation (eg, atopy or superior limbal keratoconjunctivitis). The source of these mucins in CP could be either the lacrimal apparatus or the nongoblet conjunctival epithelium, with contributions from remaining conjunctival goblet cells. Histologic studies[105] have indicated that the acinar epithelium of both the main and accessory lacrimal gland tissues contains PAS-positive granules. In addition, PAS-positive, alcian blue-positive granules containing neutral glycoproteins, sialomucin, and sulfomucin have been observed by light microscope in nongoblet conjunctival epithelial cells.[106,107] Transmission electron microscopy studies of the conjunctiva in patients with anesthetized corneas have shown similar PAS-positive vesicles just below the apical membranes of conjunctival surface cells.[108]

Transmission Electron Microscopy of Mucus—In order to further study ocular mucus in patients with CP, we performed ultrastructural analyses, using histochemical techniques, of conjunctival epithelial and surface mucus. Dr Peter Wells developed the techniques for these studies; their application to human tissue has not been previously reported. Normal human conjunctiva specimens, harvested prior to cataract surgery, were compared with specimens from patients with CP. Fresh-harvested conjunctival tissue was immersed in a fixative containing 4% glutaraldehyde and 0.1 mol/l sodium cacodylate buffer, pH 7.2. Specimens were then prepared for one of five analyses.

Cationized Ferritin. After the primary aldehyde fixation, tissue was washed with 0.05 mol/l sodium PBS, pH 7.4, and treated with 200 mol/l glycine in 0.1 mol/l sodium phosphate buffer, pH 7.4, for 30 minutes to block any unreacted aldehyde groups. Tissue was then washed with PBS and incubated with cationized ferritin (0.33 mg/ml) in PBS for 1 hour at 25°C. Controls were incubated with native horse spleen ferritin in the same manner. Following incubation with ferritin, the tissue was washed with PBS, fixed for 30 minutes with 1.5% glutaraldehyde in 0.1 mol/l sodium cacodylate buffer, washed with 0.1 mol/l sodium cacodylate, and postfixed with 1% osmium tetroxide.

Digestion with Neuraminidase. Tissue was fixed with 4% glutaraldehyde, washed with PBS, and quenched with glycine as outlined above for the cationized ferritin procedure. The tissue for neuraminidase digestion was placed in PBS, pH 5.5, containing neuraminidase, 1.25 U/ml. Control tissue was placed in PBS, pH 5.5, without enzyme. All tissue was incubated for 40 minutes at 37°C, washed with PBS, pH 7.2, and incubated with cationized ferritin, 0.33 mg/ml as outlined above.

Alcian Blue Staining. After initial fixation, conjunctival biopsies were washed with 0.1 mol/1 sodium cacodylate buffer, pH 7.2, and treated for 3 hours at 25°C with 1% alcian blue 8GX, 2% glutaraldehyde, and 0.1 mol/1 sodium cacodylate buffer, pH 6.5. Control tissue was incubated in 2% glutaraldehyde and 0.1 mol/l sodium cacodylate buffer, pH 6.5, for 3 hours at 25°C. After treatment with alcian blue, the tissue was washed with 0.1 mol/l sodium cacodylate buffer and postfixed with 1% osmium tetroxide in 0.1 mol/l sodium cacodylate.

High Iron Diamine Staining. After the primary aldehyde fixation, tissue was washed with 0.1 mol/1 sodium acetate buffer, pH 7.0, and incubated 24 hours at 25°C with 0.24% N,N-dimethyl-m-phenylene diamine hydro–chloride, 0.04% N, N-dimethyl-p-phenylene diamine hydrochloride, and 1.12% ferric chloride, pH 1.4. Control tissue was incubated 24 hours in the diamine solution, pH 1.4, without ferric chloride. After the high iron diamine incubation, the tissue was washed with 0.1 mol/l sodium acetate buffer and postfixed for 5 hours with

1% osmium tetroxide in 0.1 mol/1 sodium cacodylate.

Periodic Acid-Thiocarbohydrazide-Silver Protein. Tissue was fixed for 1 hour with glutaraldehyde as outlined above, washed with 0.1 mol/l sodium acetate buffer, pH 7.0, dehydrated with a graded series of ethanols, infiltrated with epon-araldite and acetone, and embedded in epon-araldite mixture. Following polymerization, ultrathin sections (approximately 90 nm) were cut and mounted on stainless steel grids. These sections were treated with periodic acid, thiocarbohydrazide, and silver protein (PATSP). Sections were floated on drops of 1% periodic acid for 45 minutes at 25°C, washed with distilled water, floated on drops of 0.2% thiocarbohydrazide in 20% acetic acid for 40 minutes at 25°C, rinsed with 10% acetic acid followed by a distilled water rinse, floated on drops of 1% silver protein in the dark for 30 minutes at 25°C, and washed with distilled water. All reagents were filtered through 0.2μm Millipore filters mounted in Swinnex adaptors. Control grids were processed in the same manner except that oxidization with 1% periodic acid was omitted.

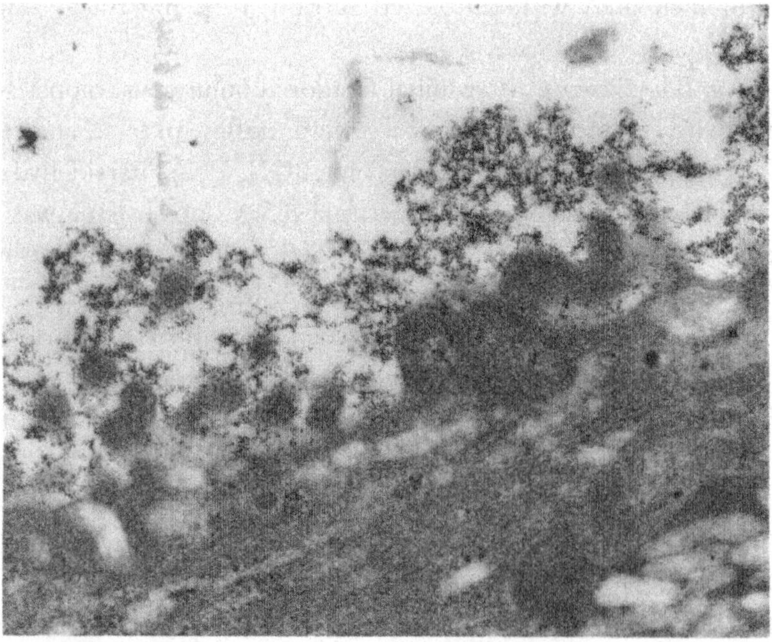

FIGURE 35: Normal conjunctiva, transmission electron microscopy, cationized ferritin (X 45,500). Uranyl acetate stain.

Postfixation and Embedding. After postfixation in 1% osmium tetroxide, tissue stained with alcian blue, cationized ferritin, and high iron diamine was dehydrated with a graded series of ethanol solutions, infiltrated with epon-araldite/acetone, and embedded in epon-araldite mixture. Thin sections (approximately 90 nm) were cut with a diamond knife mounted in an ultramicrotome. Sections cut from alcian blue or cationized ferritin blocks were stained with 2% aqueous uranyl acetate for 20 minutes. Sections cut from high iron diamine blocks were examined and photographed unstained. Transmission electron micrographs were taken with a JEM-100C electron microscope operating at 80 kV. Light microscopy of 2-μm sections was performed with a Zeiss photomicroscope using Kodak Panatomic-X film.

Analysis of Specimens. This study included four cataract patients with normal conjunctiva and five patients with CP. Ocular surface mucus in normal conjunctiva stained positively with cationized ferritin which binds to negatively charged carboxyl groups and sulfate esters (Fig 35). This staining was greatly reduced when biopsy material was incubated with neuraminidase before staining (Fig 36). This result indicated that most of the positive sites for cationized ferritin were associated with N-acetyl neuraminic acid residues in the ocular mucus. Cationized ferritin also stained ocular surface mucus in CP patients (Figs 37 and 38). Compared with normal conjunctiva, however, this staining sometimes appeared reduced or discontinuous. Alcian blue 8GX, which also stains carboxyl groups and sulfate esters, stained a layer of mucus 0.15 to 0.25 μm thick overlying the conjunctival epithelium (Fig 39). High iron diamine, which is specific for sulfate esters, stained glycocalyx and surface mucus only weakly, indicating that a small number of sulfate esters are present at the ocular surface. High iron diamine staining was similar in normal and CP conjunctiva. The PATSP technique also stained a layer of surface mucus 0.15 to 0.25 μm thick in normal conjunctiva (Fig 40), indicating that ocular mucus contains vicinal 1,2 glycols characteristic of mucins and neutral glycoproteins.

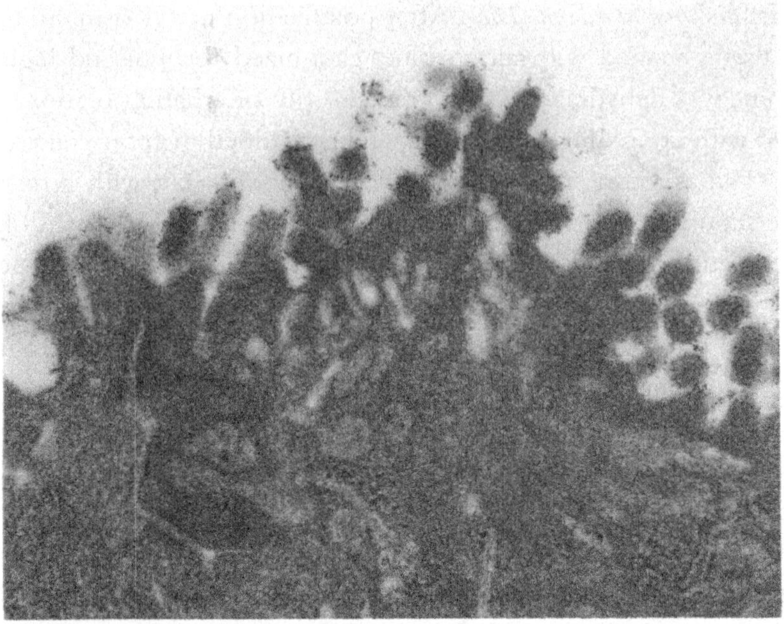

FIGURE 36: Normal conjunctiva, transmission electron microscopy, incubated with neuraminidase (1.25 U/ml). Followed by cationized ferritin (X 45,500). Uranyl acetate stain.

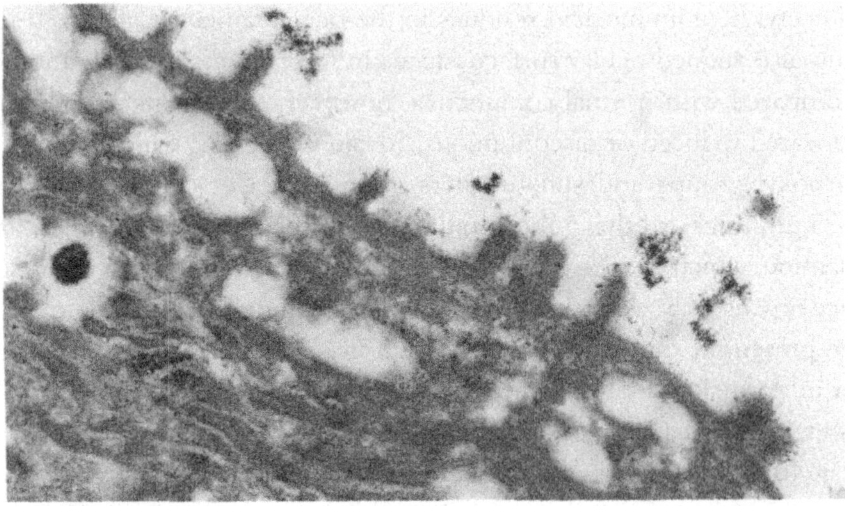

FIGURE 37: Transmission electron micrograph (X 45,500). Specimen from a CP patient successfully controlled with immunosuppressive therapy. Cationized ferritin staining.

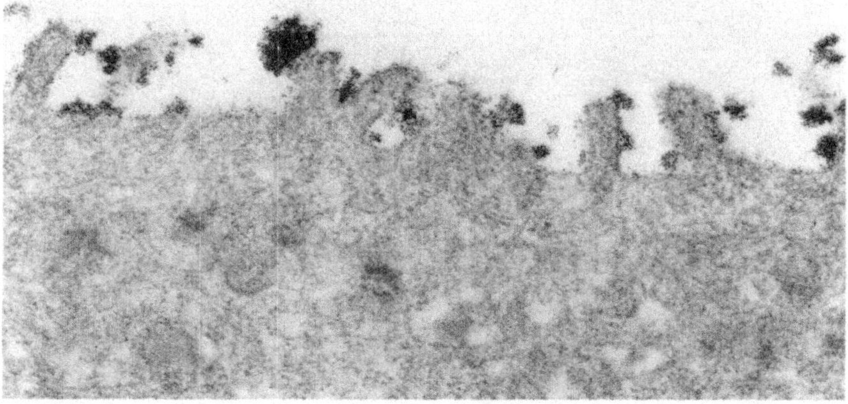

FIGURE 38: Transmission electron micrograph (X 45,500). Specimen from a CP patient successfully controlled with immunosuppressive therapy. Cationized ferritin staining.

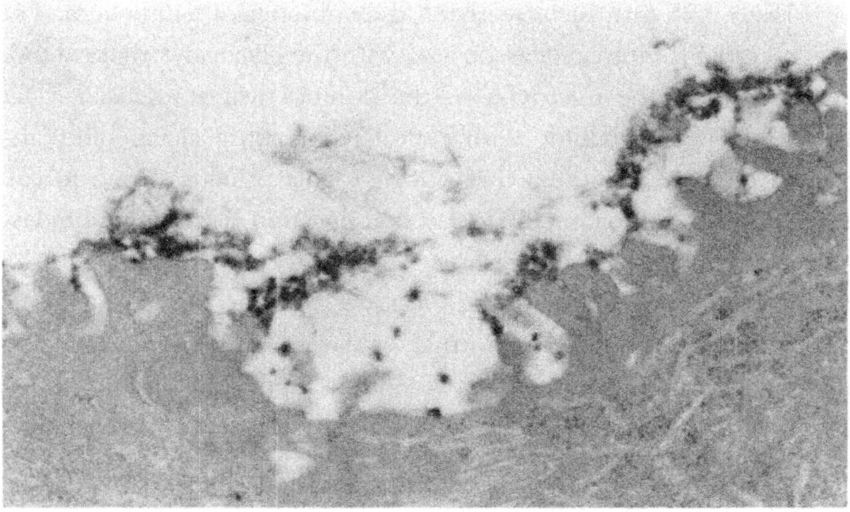

FIGURE 39: Normal conjunctiva, transmission electron microscopy, stained before embedding with alcian blue 8GX (X 35,000). Uranyl acetate staining.

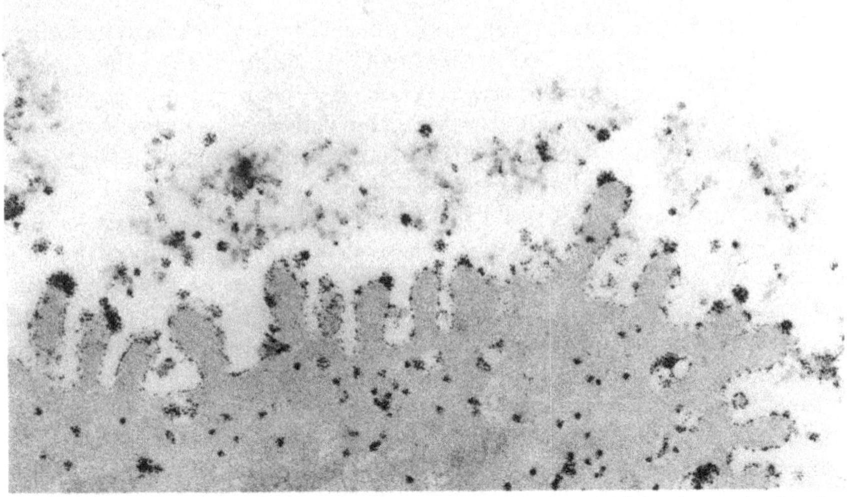

FIGURE 40: Normal conjunctiva fixed with 4% glutaraldehyde, embedded in epon-araldite, thin sectioned and stained with PATSP for vicinal l,2 glycols. Transmission electron microscopy (x 45,500).

The results of the histochemistry analyses by transmission electron microscopy suggest that human ocular mucus normally consists of a layer 0.15 to 0.25 μm thick overlying the conjunctival epithelium. The mucus material is intimately associated with the glycocalyx that extends from the tips of the microvilli of the conjunctival epithelial surface cells. Results from staining with cationized ferritin, alcian blue, and high iron diamine suggested that normal ocular mucus is rich in carboxyl groups and poor in sulfate esters. Digestion with neuraminidase confirmed that most of the carboxyl groups were associated with N-acetyl neuraminic acid (sialic acid) residues. Ocular surface mucus in CP appeared very similar to normal ocular mucus except that after staining with cationized ferritin, CP mucus appeared discontinuous. This result suggests that CP mucus contains fewer negative charges than normal mucus.

Lectins—In order to characterize the carbohydrate sidechains associated with the mucin macromolecules, we employed a panel of lectins including *Helix pomatia* agglutinin (HPA), soybean agglutinin (SBA), wheat germ agglutinin (WGA), succinylated WGA (S-WGA), peanut agglutinin (PNA), and Concanavalin A (Con-A). The carbohydrate specificities of these lectins are shown in Table XIII. Fluorescein-conjugated PNA, SBA, WGA, and Con-A have been used by others to detect goblet cell mucins in normal human conjunctiva.[109] We have also used fluorescein-conjugated lectins in light microscopic analyses of mucus in normal human conjunctiva, but we have extended these studies to biopsy specimens from CP patients, using fluorescein isothiocyanate (FITC)-conjugated lectins for light microscopy and ferritin-conjugated lectins for transmission electron microscopy.

Freshly harvested conjunctival tissue for light microscopy was placed on saline-moistened gauze and then transported to the cryostat where it was embedded in OCT compound (Tissue-Tek, Miles Laboratories) and frozen immediately at -25°C. Sections (4 μm thick) were cut, mounted on gelatin-coated glass slides, and allowed to air dry at room temperature. The sections were washed with PBS and incubated with fluorescein-conjugated lectins diluted with PBS. The slides were washed three times with PBS, coverslipped with 90% glycerol in PBS, and observed with a Zeiss Photomicroscope fitted with epi-illumination for FITC fluorescence. The slides were photographed with Kodak ASA-400 Ektachrome daylight slide film. Controls consisted of tissue sections incubated with the fluorescein-conjugated lectins mixed with the appropriate blocking sugars. Lactose (0.2 mol/1) in PBS was used to block PNA, HPA, and SBA; N,N-diacetylchitobiose (1 mmol/1) in PBS was used to block WGA and S-WGA; and α-methyl-mannose (0.2 mol/1) in PBS was used to block Con-A.

Conjunctival biopsy material for transmission electron microscopy was fixed with 4% glutaraldehyde in 0.1 mol/l sodium cacodylate buffer, washed with PBS, and quenched with glycine as outlined above for cationized ferritin. Small pieces of tissue were then incubated for 60 minutes at 25°C with ferritin-conjugated WGA, ferritin-conjugated PNA, and ferritin-conjugated SBA. All the ferritin-conjugated lectins were diluted to 25 mg/ml with PBS. Control tissue was incubated with ferritin-conjugated lectins mixed with the appropriate blocking sugar. The same blocking sugars were used for transmission EM as for light microscopy. After incubation with the lectins, tissue was washed with PBS, fixed for 30 minutes with 2.5% glutaraldehyde in 0.1 mol/l sodium cacodylate buffer, and postfixed with 1% osmium tetroxide. Tissue was dehydrated with ethanol, embedded in epon-araldite, and sectioned as outlined above for transmission electron microscope studies of mucus histochemistry.

TABLE XIII: LECTIN SPECIFICITIES

LECTIN	CARBOHYDRATE SPECIFICITY
HPA	N-acetyl-galactosamine > N-acetyl-glucosamine > galactose
SBA	N-acetyl-galactosamine > galactose
WGA	N-acetyl-glucosamine, sialic acid
S-WGA	N-acetyl-glucosamine
PNA	Galactose (1-> 3)-N-acetyl galactosamine
Con-A	Mannose > glucose > N-acetyl-glucosamine

Light microscopy of cryostat sections from CP biopsies stained with fluorescein-conjugated lectins indicated that the same carbohydrate appeared in CP mucus as in normal ocular mucus. WGA, which binds sialic acid and glucosamine residues, stained the conjunctival epithelium, surface mucus, and goblet cell granules when they were present in the biopsy specimen (Fig 41a, b, and c). WGA stained the ocular surface intensely in CP patients. S-WGA, which binds only glucosamine residues, stained conjunctival epithelium, stroma, and goblet cell granules. Both PNA, which binds galactose (1-3)-N-ace-acetyl-galactosamine residues, and HPA, which binds galactosamine, galactose, and glucosamine residues, stained goblet cell mucus granules specifically (Figs 42 and 43a and b). In CP biopsies that did not contain goblet cells, these lectins were not visualized by light microscopy. SBA, which binds galactosamine and galactose residues, stained apical conjunctival epithelial cells, goblet cell granules, and ocular surface mucus (Fig 44a and b). Con-A which stains mannose, was negative for ocular mucus, as was expected since most mucins do not contain mannose residues in the oligosaccharide sidechains.

Staining of surface mucus was checked by transmission electron microscopy using ferritin-conjugated WGA. This lectin appeared to bind to a layer of mucus material, 0.15 to 0.25 µm thick, at the conjunctival surface. The mucus material stained with WGA appeared similar in thickness and distribution to the mucus material stained with cationized ferritin, alcian blue, and PATSP. Ferritin-conjugated PNA did not stain surface mucus at the transmission electron microscopic level.

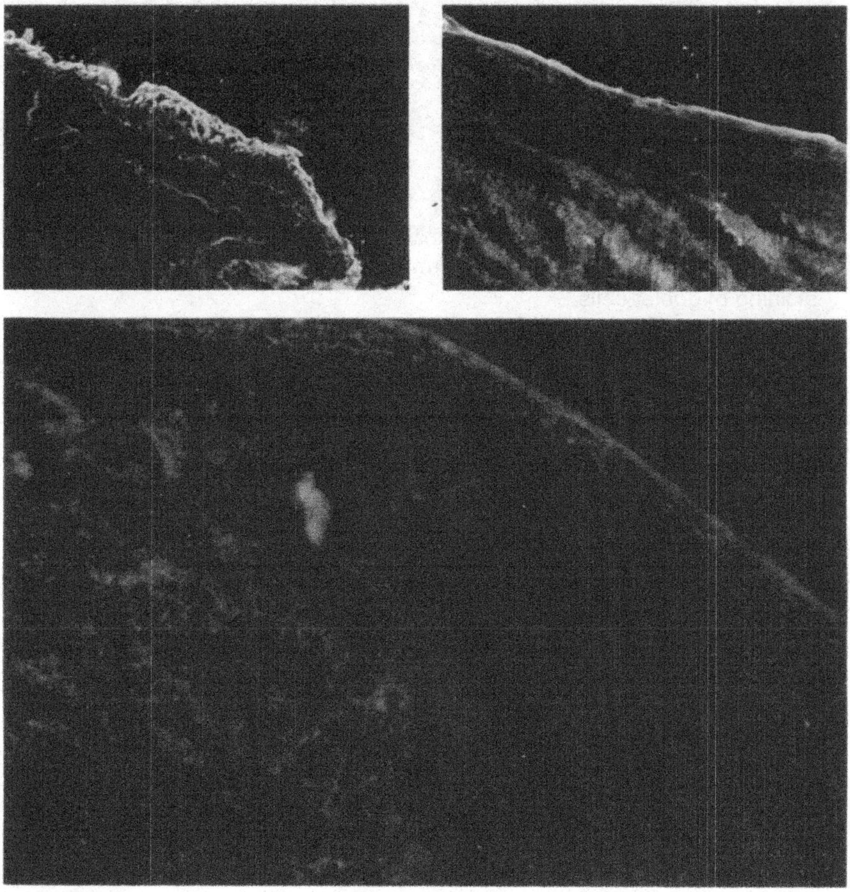

<u>FIGURE 41:</u> a: IF (X 160). Normal conjunctiva, WGA. Note positive reaction (staining) of conjunctival epithelium as well as layer of mucus at epithelial surface. b: IF (x 60). Active C P conjunctival specimen. Note intense staining of surface of specimen which correlates with surface mucus mat. Epithelial cells also stain. c: Section stained with WCA previously incubated with diacetylchitobiose. The absence of surface fluorescence demonstrates specificity of FITC conjugated WGA.

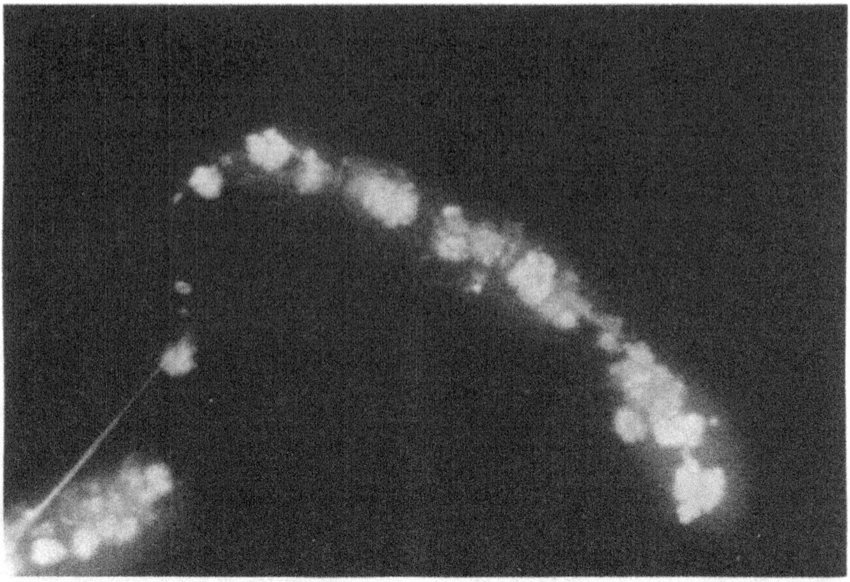

FIGURE 42: IF, PNA (x 160). Normal human conjunctiva. Note intense staining of goblet cells.

These results with lectins indicate that ocular mucus, in both patients with CP and individuals with normal conjunctiva, is rich in N-acetyl glucosamine, galactose, and N-acetyl-galactosamine residues. In some CP patients WGA stained with ocular surface intensely at the light microscopic level, suggesting that these patients possessed an elevated amount of surface mucus rich in sialic acid or N-acetyl-glucosamine residues. Since major differences between the staining patterns or normal and CP ocular mucus were not observed, it is presumed that the remaining goblet cells in CP patients add glucosamine, galactosamine, and galactose to the mucin polypeptide backbone in a normal manner, and that saccharide addition to the mucin macromolecules is not deficient in CP.

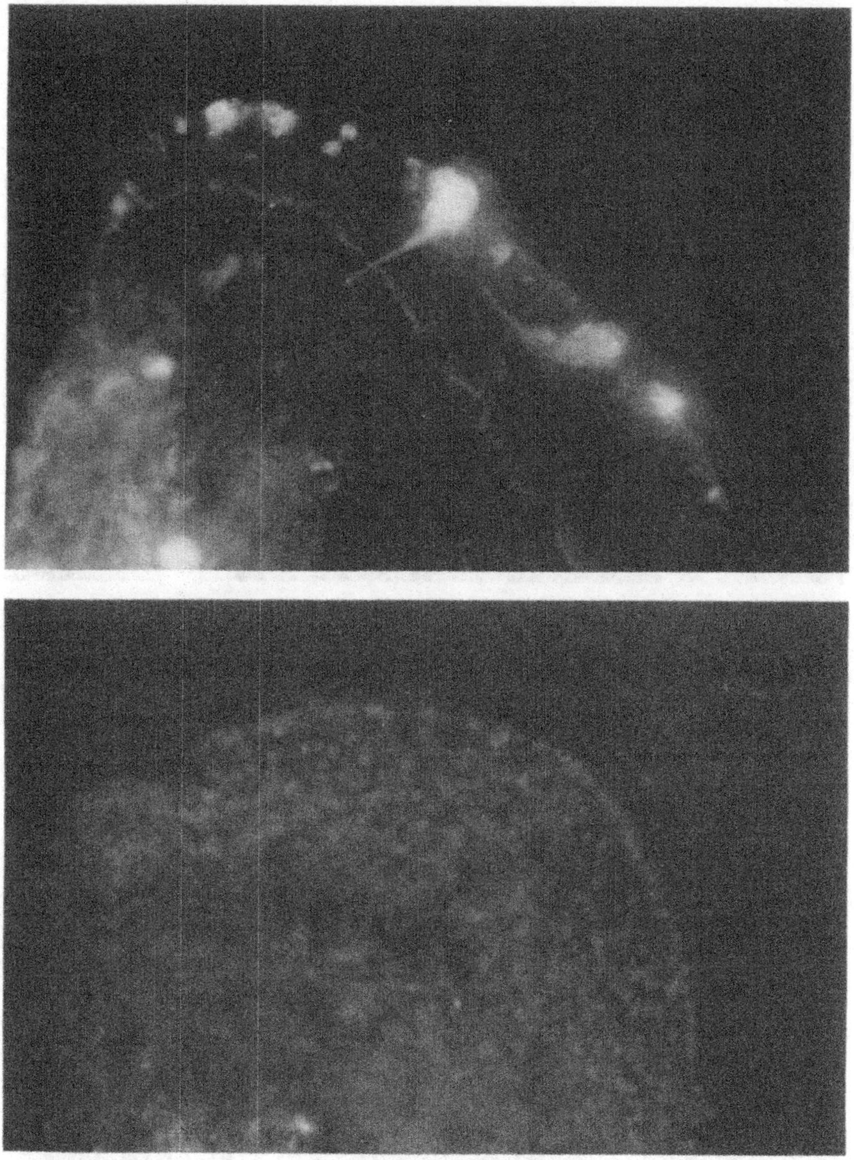

FIGURE 43: a: IF, PNA (x 160). Conjunctival specimen from patient with active CP. Note staining of goblet cells present in this specimen. b: Section stained with PNA previously incubated with lactose. Blocking of staining demonstrates specificity of FITC conjugated PNA.

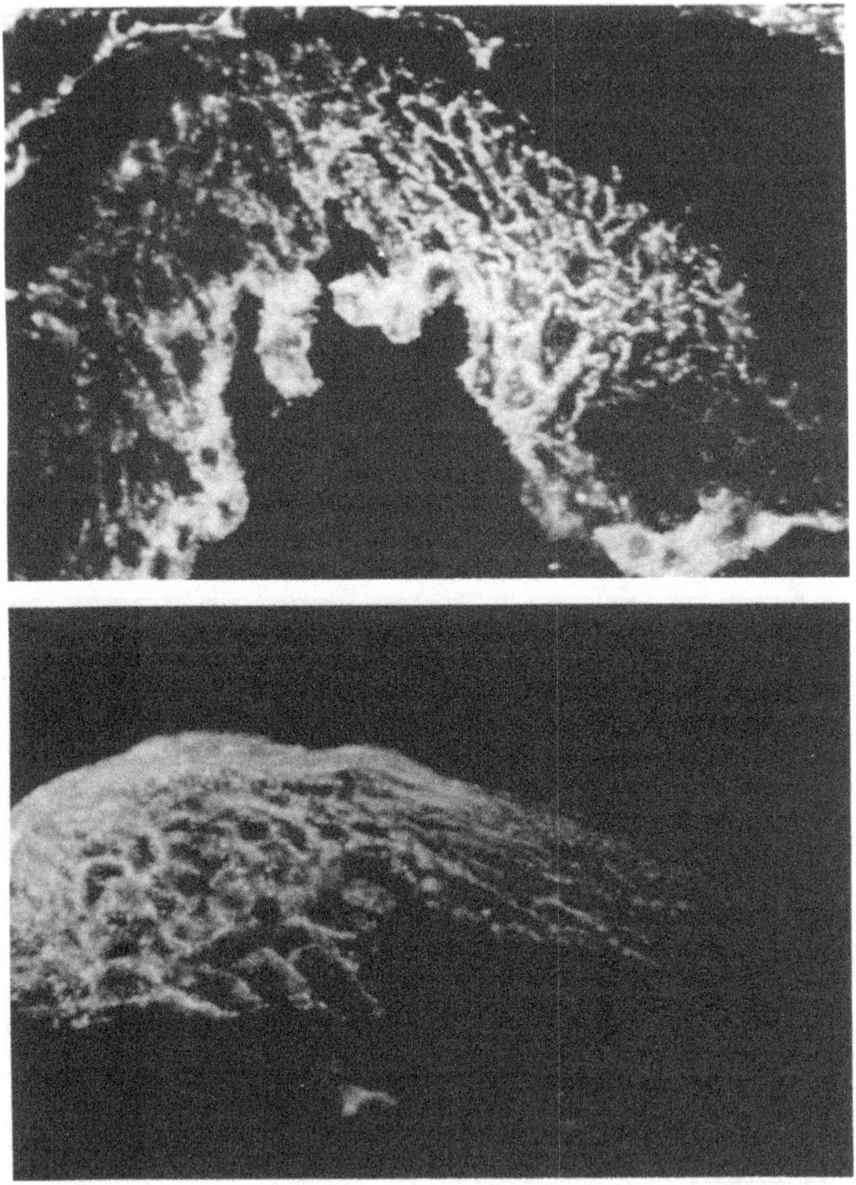

FIGURE 44: a: IF (x 160), normal conjunctiva, fluoresceinated SBA. Note staining of epithelial cells, granules within goblet cell, and surface mucus. b: IF (x 150) SBA. Specimen from patient with active CP. Note positive staining of epithelial cells as well as a thin surface mat, most probably mucus.

IMMUNOPATHOLOGY

Immunofluorescence

We chose to perform all our IF and immunoperoxidase studies on fresh, snap-frozen specimens embedded in cryostat embedding compound and sectioned on a cryostat microtome. We chose this technique because we noted some loss of sensitivity, presumably from antigen site alterations, when we employed fixation techniques, including St Marie's fixation. All specimens were snap-frozen in liquid nitrogen, embedded in OCT, and stored at -70°C until sectioning, staining, and analysis within 6 weeks of harvesting. IF techniques were used for all specimens. The panel of antisera we employ is shown in Table XIV, along with our typical working dilution for each.

TABLE XIV

ANTISERUM (IgG FRACTION)	WORKING DILUTION
Rabbit anti-human IgA	1:16
Rabbit anti-human IgD	1:8
Rabbit anti-human IgE	1:8
Rabbit anti-human IgG	1:30
Rabbit anti-human IgM	1:8
Rabbit anti-human C_3	1:4
Rabbit anti-human C_4	1:4
Rabbit anti-human albumen	1:30
Rabbit anti-human fibrinogen	1:16

TABLE XV: IF AT THE BMZ OF CONJUNCTIVAL SPECIMENS FROM 130 PATIENTS WITH CP

ANTISERUM	NO. POSITIVE SPECIMENS (%)	NO. SPECIMENS POSITIVE FOR ONLY ONE ANTISERUM
IgA	55 (42)	9
IgG	53 (41)	11
IgM	21 (16)	3
IgD	13 (10)	3
IgE	29 (22)	1
C_3	31 (24)	3
C_4	32 (25)	2

Antiserum specificity is checked by Ouchterlony analysis, by preanalysis blocking experiments, and by postabsorption experiments documenting loss of specific staining reaction by prior absorption with specific antigen (eg, IgA) coupled to Sepharose 4B beads. For conjugation of protein antigen to Sepharose beads, we used standard procedures. Briefly, purified protein was dialyzed in 0.1 mol/1 sodium bicarbonate overnight at 4°C with stirring, using 80 times as much sodium bicarbonate as protein solution; the protein was typically in solution in PBS at an approximate concentration of 30 to 40 mg/ml. Three grams of cyanogen bromide-activated Sepharose 4B beads were allowed to swell, at 4°C, in 0.1 mol/1 sodium bicarbonate buffer, pH 9.0. The beads were soaked in a small, coarse sintered glass filter on a side-arm vacuum flask, in 50 ml of 0.001 mol/1 hydrochloric acid for 15 minutes, with subsequent vacuum application to the flask and multiple hydrochloric acid washes of the beads. The beads were then washed with 50-ml aliquots of 0.1 mol/1 sodium bicarbonate. The beads were added to the protein solution in a small beaker with a stir bar, and incubated with stirring at room temperature for 4 hours, or at 4°C overnight. The beads were then washed in the sintered glass vacuum .filter, first with 0.2 mol/1 glycine (pH 2.2), then with 0.1 mol/1 sodium bicarbonate (pH 8.0), followed by three successive similar alternating glycine/sodium bicarbonate washes. Finally, each sample was washed once with 0.5 mol/1 sodium phosphate buffer (pH 7.0), then twice with PBS. Absorption of antisera was achieved by incubating these conjugated beads with the antiserum in a 1:1 proportion for 1 hour at 37°C with shaking, followed by subsequent incubation at 4°C overnight. The procedure ended with centrifugation at 2000 rpm, supernatant harvesting, and analysis of supernatant with specific antigen to check for completeness of absorption. Similar coupling and absorption strategies were employed for any antiserum with unacceptably high background staining reactions.

Our IF studies require scrupulous attention to tissue processing and sectioning to maintain the highest possible level of natural morphology. We were usually disappointed by the handling and analysis of conjunctival specimens by nonophthalmic pathology and immunopathology laboratories. The technicians in such laboratories are unfamiliar with the delicacy of conjunctiva and are uncomfortable working with such tiny, delicate specimens.

To avoid artifacts, it was essential to minimize thawing of tissue during handling. The specimen embedded in OCT compound was quickly transferred from the -70°C Revco freezer to the cryostat unit, and quickly affixed to a precooled chuck on which had been placed a small amount of fresh OCT compound. Sections were then cut in the cryostat microtome at a thickness of 4 µm, and picked up onto glass slides that had previously been coated with gelatin to prevent tissue loss during washing and staining. Slides may be air dried with a fan for 30 minutes and then may be stained, but we found that less tissue washed off if the slides were stored overnight before being stained.

We found it crucial to use the highest quality fluorescein- or rhodamine-labeled antisera available to ensure optimal tissue analysis. The antisera should be highly reactive with the specific antigen, yet should display a minimum amount of background staining. The best reagents for tissue staining are IgG fractions of fluorescein- or rhodamine-labeled antisera with two to four molecules of label per molecule of antibody protein. Fluorescein (FITC)- or rhodamine (TRITC) tetramethylrhodamine isothiocyanate-conjugated IgG fractions are available from a number of companies (Cappel, Meloy, Bionetics, Cedarlane). Most commercial conjugates are lyophilized and are usually restored with distilled water unless diluent is supplied by the manufacturer.

We usually relied on the conjugated IgG fractions of antisera from Cappel Laboratories and found their quality control to be reliable. Stock aliquots of the antisera were pipetted into vials as soon as they were received and were stored at -20°C until use. Optimal dilutions of the conjugates were determined by use of known positive and negative controls. Working dilutions for indirect IF were usually greater than for direct IF, due to an amplification effect.

Antisera were diluted in 0.02 mol/l PBS with 1% bovine serum albumin(except for rabbit anti-human albumin, which was diluted in PBS alone). Two drops of 0.05% sodium azide were added and the antisera were sterile filtered. These solutions could then be stored at 4°C. Conjugates were centrifuged before use (8000 X g for 15 minutes) to remove aggregates that may have formed during storage.

Slides to be stained were air dried for 20 minutes after removal from the freezer. They were then washed in PBS for 10 minutes to remove unbound protein. The slide was then gently blotted around the specimen to remove PBS, and one drop (20 to 50 μl) of appropriately diluted conjugate antiserum, warmed to room temperature, was applied to cover the tissue. The slides were incubated in a moist, level chamber for 30 minutes at room temperature. Excess stain was drained following the incubation, and the slides are washed, three times, in fresh PBS for 10 minutes. The slide around the specimen was then dried and a coverslip and modified mountant, which helps prevent fluorescent fading during the fluorescence microscopy, were added. The rapid fading of the fluorochrome FITC in fluorescence microscopy can be a nuisance, particularly when one wishes to document results by fluorescence photomicroscopy. The modified mountant that we used, developed by Mr Kevin McNamee of Carl Zeiss, LTD, London, inhibits fading even after 20 minutes of continuous exposure to the activating fluorescence light source. This mountant was composed of 0.1% p-phenylenedimine in glycerol and phosphate-bicarbonate buffer.

Our fluorescence microscopy was conducted on our Zeiss Photomic III fluorescence microscope with a vertical illuminator III RS for epifluorescence, and band pass (BP) excitation filter (450 to 490 nm) and (520 to 560 nm) BP barrier filter for fluorescein conjugates, and a 515 to 560 nm BP excitation filter and a long wave pass barrier filter blocking all wavelengths below 590 nm for rhodamine conjugates. Photographic documentation of results was achieved through the on-plane spot metering automatic exposure device. The results of our IF studies appear in Table XV. The most notable feature of these data is the finding that 25% of the specimens (32 of 130) had a single immunoreactant detectable by IF technique. "Standard" IF antisera panels (antisera against IgG, IgA, IgM, and C_3) would have missed BMZ positivity in 5% of the specimens that were found to be positive by IF technique.

Fig 45 shows the typical continuous, homogeneous, thin, apple-green, IF-positive line at the conjunctival epithelial BMZ in a positive CP specimen; the antiserum in this instance was reactive with IgA. We have never seen this appearance in our analysis of well over 100 specimens of normal conjunctiva or of conjunctiva from patients with other inflammatory disorders (Mooren's ulcer, systemic lupus erythematosus, rosacea blepharoconjunctivitis, atopic blepharoconjunctivitis, staphylococcal keratoconjunctivitis). The intensity of BMZ staining in CP specimens varied from patient to patient. Some specimens exhibited a discontinuous pattern. A few specimens showed a granular instead of a homogeneous pattern.

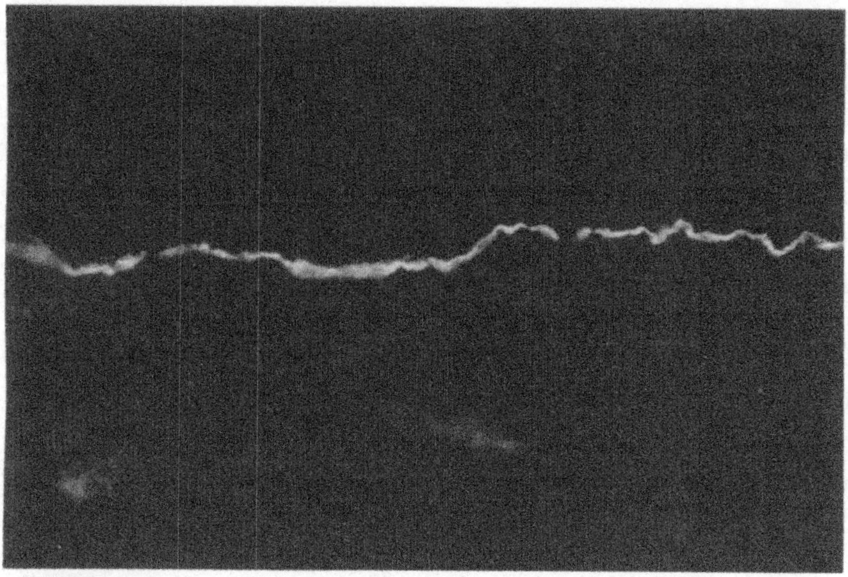

FIGURE 45: IF (x 160). Fluoresceinated anti-human IgA. Note intense (4+) positivity at epithelial BMZ.

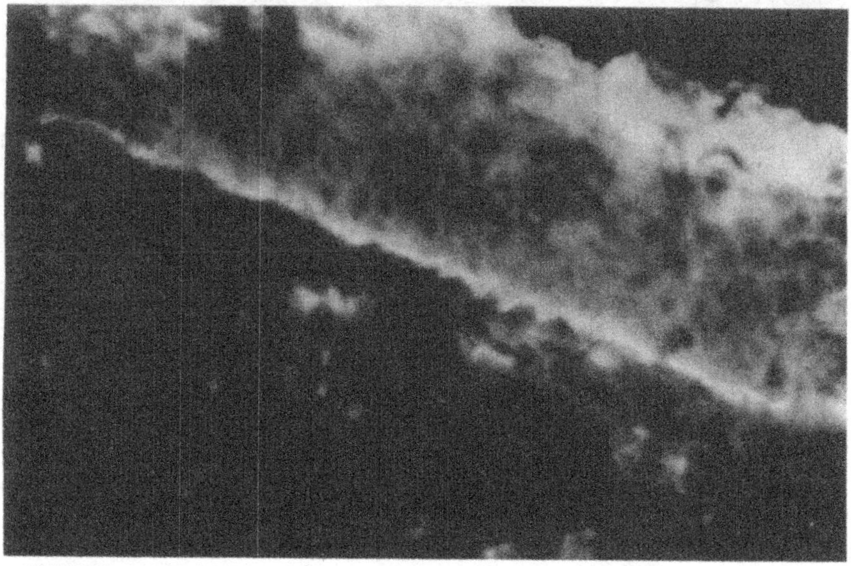

FIGURE 46: IF (X 160). Fluoresceinated anti-human IgA. Note, in addition to BMZ positivity, 4+ positivity of superficial epithelial cells.

Epithelial positivity (Fig 46) for one or more immunoreactant (most commonly IgA) was seen in 32% of the specimens. This feature was usually found in patients with the most extreme (4+) degree of ocular inflammation at the time of biopsy. We could not correlate this finding or the type of immunoreactant present at the BMZ with subsequent response to therapy. Nor could we correlate therapeutic response with presence or absence of immunoreactant deposition in conjunctival vessel walls (Fig 47).

Fourteen of the 130 specimens were negative by direct IF (10.8%). Attempts to amplify subtle, low density immunoreactant reactivity at the BMZ through indirect IF techniques did not increase our ability to detect positive specimens. Application of an immunoperoxidase technique to the IF-negative specimens, however, did result in enhanced sensitivity, *without* loss of specificity; negative controls remained negative by the immunoperoxidase technique.

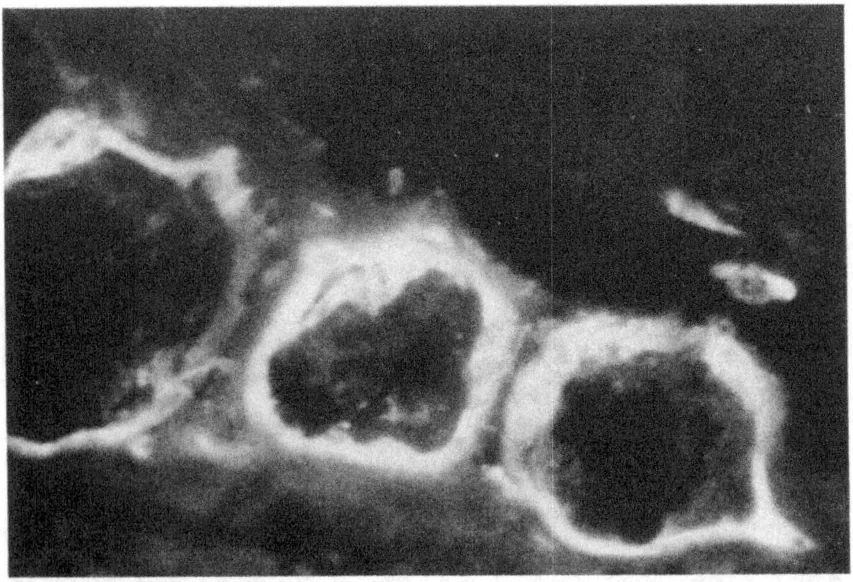

FIGURE 47: IF (x 500). Fluoresceinated anti-human C_3. Note staining of vessel walls.

Immunoperoxidase

Though substantially more labor-intensive (and hence more expensive), the ABC immunoperoxidase technique is approximately 1000 times more sensitive than the IF technique. We therefore have consistently used the ABC technique on specimens from patients who clinically appeared to have CP, but for whom the IF analysis of conjunctiva was negative. Briefly, cryostat sections were air dried for 20 minutes and the tissue was then prefixed with 100% acetone for 10 minutes. The slides were then air dried at room temperature and incubated with diluted normal serum for 20 minutes. They were then incubated with the primary antibody for 1 hour at room temperature and washed twice, 10 minutes each time, with PBS. Endogenase peroxidase blocking was accomplished by a 30-minute incubation with 0.3% hydrogen peroxide in PBS. The slides were then washed with PBS for 10 minutes and incubated with biotinylated antibody solution for 30 minutes to 2 hours, depending on the appropriate incubation time as judged by preliminary experiments in staining intensity. Three subsequent 10-minute washes with PBS were followed by incubation with the ABC reagent for 40 minutes. Slides were then washed with PBS twice for 10 minutes, and the peroxidase substrate was prepared. Ten milligrams of 3-amino-9-ethylcarbacole was dissolved in 2.5 ml N,N-dimethylformamide. Fifty milliliters of 0.1 mol/l sodium acetate buffer, pH 5.0, and 30 µm of hydrogen peroxide (50%) were then added, and the solution filtered. The slides were then incubated in a Coplin jar with the peroxidase substrate. Staining was monitored visually, and typically developed within 5 to 15 minutes. The slides were then fixed with 4% formalin and 0.1 mol/l sodium acetate buffer for 5 to 10 minutes. They were washed with 1% glacial acetic acid, counterstained with Gill's No 3 hematoxylin for 10 seconds, and washed with water until the effluent was clear. The slides were then washed in 1% acetic acid until the nuclei were well stained, and were subsequently washed four more times with water. They were then dipped in saturated lithium carbonate solution, washed with water (four or five changes over 20 minutes), and cover-slipped with Gelvatol.

The results of ABC peroxidase analysis of IF-negative specimens from CP subjects (Fig 48) are shown in Table XVI.

I am currently following 12 patients whose clinical ocular features were compatible with the diagnosis of stage II CP, but for whom both IF and immunoperoxidase analyses were negative. Nine of these patients are atopic, and three have acne rosacea. Treatment of these conditions has controlled conjunctival inflammation, but long-term observation for progressive conjunctival cicatrization (and rebiopsy for immunopathologic analysis) will presumably disclose whether or not these cases have been appropriately classified as not representing CP.

I have been unable to correlate therapeutic response to individual chemotherapeutic agents with the BMZ immunopathologic features of the biopsy specimens from CP patients. I wondered if T-cell subset analysis would provide such a correlation.

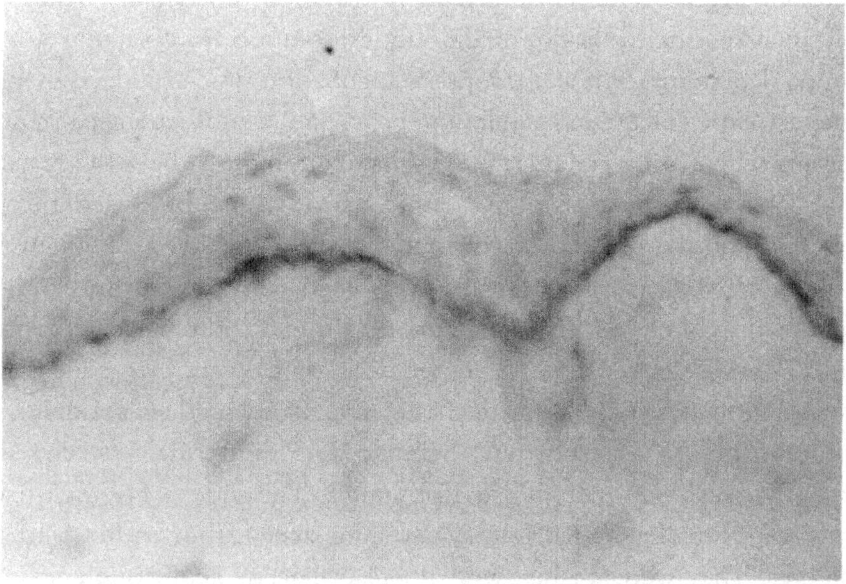

FIGURE 48: Immunoperoxidase-ABC (X 160). Anti-human IgG. Note positivity at epithelial BMZ in this specimen which was negative by IF technique.

T-Cell Subsets

Characterization of lymphocyte subsets at the site of inflammatory reactions can provide valuable information regarding the pathogenesis of a disease process. The development of monoclonal antibodies against human T-cells and T-cell subsets has made it possible to differentiate the functional subsets of human lymphocytes in tissue sections. I applied this technology, employing the immunoperoxidase ABC technique, to the infiltrating lymphocytes in inflammatory conjunctival lesions associated with CP. An initial pilot portion of this study was conducted in collaboration with Drs Leslie Fujikawa and Atul Bhan.

Specimens were obtained from the inferior bulbar conjunctiva of 10 patients with active CP and of 10 age- and sex-matched control patients undergoing cataract surgery. The specimens were snap-frozen, embedded in OCT compound, and stored at -70°C for 2 to 12 weeks until analysis.

We used monoclonal antibodies that react with T lymphocyte surface antigens. In brief, the monoclonal antibodies anti-T1 and anti-T3 react with all peripheral T-cells and intensely with 10% of thymocytes. Anti-T6 antibody reacts with 70% of thymocytes, but not with peripheral T-cells. Anti-T6 antibody also stains Langerhans' cells in the skin and lymph nodes. Anti-T4 antibody reacts with about 60% of circulating T-cells and defines inducer/helper T-cells. Anti-T8 antibody reacts with about 30% of circulating T-cells and defines suppressor/cytotoxic T cells. We also used another monoclonal antibody, anti-T4B (clone No SC1-12T4D11), which stains the same cell population as anti-T4, but more intensely. Anti-T10 antibody reacts with most thymocytes, a significant proportion of activated T-cells, and only a minority of peripheral T-cells. Anti-T10 antibody also stains a subpopulation of B cells and the cytoplasm of plasma cells in tissue sections, and is therefore not specific for T-cells.

TABLE XVI: IMMUNOPEROXIDASE ABC ANALYSIS OF IF-NEGATIVE CONJUNCTIVAL SPECIMENS FROM 14 CP SUSPECTS

ANTISERUM	NO. POSITIVE SPECIMENS (%)	NO. SPECIMENS POSITIVE FOR ONLY ONE ANTISERUM
IgA	8 (57)	4
IgG	9 (64)	0
IgM	4 (28)	2
IgD	3 (21)	1
IgE	0 (0)	0
C_3	4 (28)	2
C_4	3 (21)	1

Anti-Ia monoclonal antibodies (anti-11 and anti-I2) react with a nonpolymorphic region of human Ia-like antigens (HLA.DR) and stain a wide variety of cells including activated T-cells, macrophages, Langerhans' cells, and endothelial cells. Anti-IgM monoclonal antibody was used to identify B cells with surface or cytoplasmic IgM.

A four-step immunoperoxidase technique employing peroxidase-anti-peroxidase complexes was used. In brief, frozen 4 μm sections were fixed in acetone, incubated with ascitic fluid containing the monoclonal antibodies, and then incubated with rabbit anti-mouse immunoglobulins and peroxidase-rabbit-anti-peroxidase reagent. Sections were stained with 3-amino-9-ethylcarbazole, which gives a red-brown product.

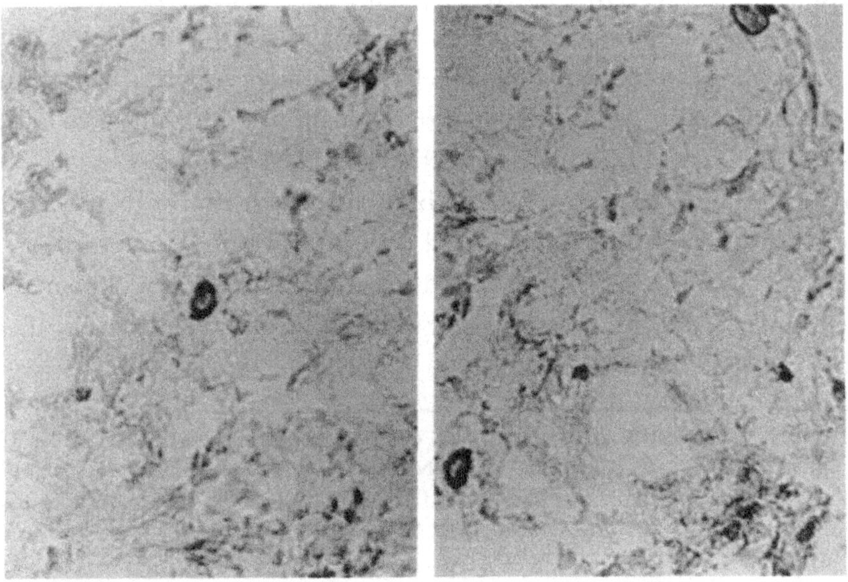

FIGURE 49: Immunoperoxidase-ABC (X 250). Normal human conjunctiva. Left panel, anti-T4 monoclonal antibody, detecting helper T-cells. One positive cell is seen . Right panel, anti-T8 antibody, detecting suppressor cells. Four positive cells are seen.

Monoclonal antibodies anti-T1, anti-T3, anti-T4, anti-T4B, and anti-T8 stained the periphery of specific cells in a manner compatible with staining of the lymphocyte membrane. Together, these antibodies stained most of the lymphocytes in the specimens, indicating that most of the lymphocytes were T-cells. Anti-IgM antibody produced peripheral staining of cells, in a pattern similar to that obtained with small B lymphocytes in primary follicles and the mantle zone of secondary follicles in lymph nodes.

In most of the specimens the stained cells in the substantia propria were T10+ plasma cells. Few cells stained with anti-T4 antibodies (which define inducer/helper T-cells); more were stained with an anti-T8 antibody (which defines suppressor/cytotoxic T-cells) (Fig 49). These suppressor/cytotoxic cells were found under the epithelium, the significance of which is not clear. T8+ cells were also found in and adjacent to the epithelium. There was little or no staining with anti-IgM antibody, indicating that few B cells with IgM were present in these normal specimens.

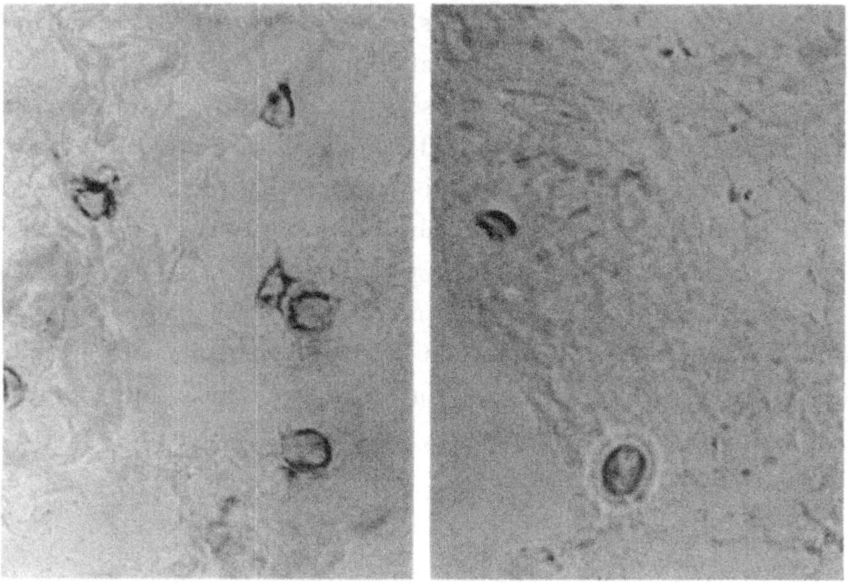

FIGURE 50: Immunoperoxidase-ABC (X 160). CP conjunctiva, left panel, anti-T4, six positive cells; right panel, anti-T8, two positive cells.

The cytoplasm of large cells with dendritic processes scattered in the epithelium stained diffusely with anti-T6 antibody, and these were considered to be Langerhans' cells. No lymphocytes or other conjunctival cells stained with this antibody.

Anti-Ia antibodies stained a few large cells (Langerhans' cells) in normal conjunctival epithelium. Staining in the substantia propria was restricted primarily to endothelial cells of blood vessels and a few cells in the stroma considered to be fibrohistiocytic cells.

In all specimens of conjunctiva from patients with CP, a cellular infiltrate was imposed on the cellular profile for normal conjunctiva. T4+ (inducer/helper) and T8+ (suppressor/cytotoxic) cells made up almost all of the mononuclear infiltrate, with T4+ cells forming by far the major component. The T4+ cells occurred in the infiltrate, in groups around blood vessels, and scattered in the substantia propria near the epithelium (Fig 50). These inducer/helper cells may play an important role in the generation of autoantibodies and in the pathogenesis of the lesions.

A few B cells stained with anti-IgM antibody were scattered in all CP specimens and were sometimes present in aggregates. Numbers of plasma cells, shown by anti-T10 antibody, were elevated. They were either scattered throughout the substantia propria or in aggregate. Langerhans' cells, defined by anti-T6 antibody, were increased both in the epithelium and in the substantia propria. Most Ia+ cells, which included lymphocytes, large cells (fibrohistiocyte cells), and endothelial cells, were located in the substantia propria.

The discrepancy between the numbers of cells stained with T4+ and T8+ suggests that a defect in immunoregulation, with an imbalance in the relative numbers and/or activity of inducer and suppressor cells may account for the genesis, or at least for the progression, of conjunctival pathology in CP.

Circulating Autoantibodies

We determined, by indirect IF, the presence or absence of three autoantibodies in all 130 of our patients with CP. RF (IgM) and ANA determinations were performed by our hospital laboratory in the usual way. Anti-BMZ antibody determinations were performed by using normal human conjunctiva as the substrate and fluoresceinated rabbit anti-human immunoglobulin (Cappel Laboratories) as the secondary antiserum.

Nineteen patients had detectable RF; they all had unequivocal rheumatoid arthritis; the RF titer in this group ranged from 1:64 to 1:1024. The 59 patients who showed positive reaction to ANA exhibited a homogeneous ANA staining pattern; the titer ranged from 1:32 to 1:512. Three patients in this group were diagnosed as having lupus erythematosus. Anti-BMZ, found in the sera of the 26 patients, occurred at consistently low titers with a range of 1:20 to 1:80.

Circulating immune complex determinations were done on 30 sera from patients with active CP in a commercial laboratory, employing C1q binding and Raji cell assays. None of the specimens contained detectable circulating immune complexes.

HLA *Typing*

HLA typing was performed in 30 patients by a commercial tissue typing laboratory. The results are shown in Table XVII.

The HLA phenotypic frequencies found in our study population were compared with the frequency distributions in the normal control "at large" population typed on a continuing basis by the tissue typing laboratory. Probability values were computed by using Fisher's exact probabilities from the distribution of the chi-square, with application of the Yates correction to the data analysis. We did not find HLA phenotypic frequencies in our study group of 30 CP patients which differed significantly from the standard reference frequencies. Mondino previously reported that HLA-Bl2 was associated with CP in his study population.[54] We were previously unable to confirm such an association,[2] and could not confirm it in this study, either.

MICROBIOLOGY—CULTURES OF MEIBUM

Our microbiologic findings were as follows. Eight of the 130 CP patients had bacterial keratitis at the time of initial referral, and 3 others developed bacterial keratitis while under our care. *Staphylococcus aureus* was isolated in nine of these cases; there was one case each of *Proteus mirabilis*, *Pseudomonas aeruginosa*, and *Serratia marcesens.*

Cultures of meibum disclosed *S aureus* and *Staphylococcus epidermis* in 9 of the 11 cases. All 11 patients were being treated with topical dexamethasone phosphate and erythromycin ointment for conjunctival inflammation and epitheliopathy at the time the microbial keratitis developed. While data support the idea that CP patients are "at risk" for microbial keratitis, they suggest that the significant risk factors are epithelial pathology, and abuse of broad-spectrum antibiotics and steroids.

BIOCHEMISTRY

Mucus Analysis by SDS—Polyacrylamide Gel Electrophoresis

The precorneal tear film is composed of three layers; an innermost mucin layer, a middle aqueous layer, and an outermost lipid layer. The innermost mucin layer is thought to be secreted by the conjunctival goblet cells, with contributions from nongoblet conjunctival epithelial cells and cells of the lacrimal gland. Ocular mucus ensures the even spread of aqueous tears over the cornea and conjunctiva. It lubricates the lids and anterior surface of the eye during blinking and may also function as a macromolecular barrier against invading microorganisms.

We studied the glycoprotein compositions of mucus from eyes of patients with CP and controls (normal individuals and patients with atopic conjunctivitis, meibomianitis, superior limbic keratoconjunctivitis, and blepharitis). As noted above, the proposal by several authors that CP and Stevens-Johnson syndrome are mucin deficiency, dry-eye syndromes is supported by histologic studies that show reduced numbers of conjunctival goblet cells in patients with these diseases. Paradoxically, thick mucus strands are often noted in the inferior fornix of patients with CP and Stevens-Johnson syndrome. Previous studies[110,111] concerning the glycoprotein composition of human ocular mucus have utilized pooled ocular mucus from normal individuals. We collected and analyzed, by sodium dodecyl sulfate (SDS)-gradient polyacrylamide gel electrophoresis, individual mucus samples from the eyes of normal individuals and patients with CP, Stevens-Johnson syndrome, and other inflammatory eye disorders. The study was performed in our laboratory in collaboration with Dr Peter Wells.

Ocular mucus samples were harvested from the eyes of 4 normal individuals and from 19 patients with CP, 4 with Stevens-Johnson syndrome, and 11 with inflammatory eye diseases. Mucus samples were collected from the inferior fornix with a sterile plastic tube, 2.0 mm in diameter. The samples were transferred to 1.5-ml microcentrifuge tubes containing sterile distilled water. Mucus samples from the right and left eyes of patients were collected and analyzed separately, and no samples were pooled. Less mucus was available from the eyes of normal individuals, however, so that the mucus threads taken from both eyes in four to six morning collections had to be pooled to provide enough material for assay. All mucus samples were stored at -70°C until assay.

Mucus samples were washed in distilled water and centrifuged (2000 x g for 15 minutes) to pellet the water-insoluble mucus. Samples were then transferred to tared 1.5-ml microcentrifuge tubes and centrifuged again with distilled water to remove water-soluble proteins. The supernates were aspirated with fine-tipped glass pipets, and the remaining mucus pellets were dried in the tared tubes at room temperature in a sterile laminar flow cabinet. They were then weighed and dissolved in gel electrophoresis sample buffer containing 8 mol/1 urea, 2% SDS, and 5% 2-mercaptoethanol. The samples were heated (90°C for 30 minutes) to complete the solubilization of the mucus.

The standard proteins for molecular weight calibration of the gels were Bio-Rad Laboratories' high-molecular-weight markers, myosin, β-galactosidase, phosphorylase A, bovine serum albumin, and ovalbumin. They were dissolved in the same sample buffer with 0.004% bromophenol blue as a tracking dye. Polyacrylamide gradient gels(% to 16%, 7.5 X 7.5 cm) were purchased precast from Pharmacia, Inc. The gels were pre-electrophoresed for 1 hour at 70 V constant voltage with 0.1 mol/1 sodium phosphate buffer, pH 7.0, containing 0.1% SDS in the upper and lower reservoirs. Samples (30 µl) were then loaded onto the gels and electrophoresis was carried out at a constant 75 V. Electrophoresis was stopped 45 minutes after the tracking dye had migrated off the gel onto the lower reservoir.

The gels were then immersed in 7% acetic acid. Lanes containing the high-molecular-weight standards were cut from the gels and stained with 0.25% Coomassie brilliant blue R-250, while the lanes containing mucus samples were stained either by a PAS technique or with 0.5% alcian blue 8GX in 3% acetic acid. Gels stained with alcian blue were destained with 7% acetic acid for 5 to 10 days.

For PAS staining, the gel was washed with 7% acetic acid at 4°C, reacted with 0.2% periodic acid for 45 to 50 minutes at 4°C, washed with distilled water at 4°C, and then stained with Schiffs reagent for 60 to 90 minutes at room temperature with constant agitation. After the pink-magenta bands appeared on a clear background, the gels were washed with distilled water and stored at 4°C in 7% acetic acid. Stained gels were transilluminated with a lightbox and photographed with 35-mm Kodak Technical Pan film.

Conjunctival biopsy specimens for diagnostic purposes were harvested from several of the patients with CP, Stevens-Johnson syndrome, and other types of ocular inflammation. The biopsies were taken from the limbal conjunctiva at either the 3 o'clock or the 9 o'clock position after administration of topical proparacaine and subconjunctival xylocaine. Biopsies were fixed immediately in Karnovsky's fixative (1% paraformaldehyde, 1.25% glutaraldehyde, 0.13% sucrose, and 25 mmol/1 sodium phosphate in 150 mmol/1 sodium cacodylate) for 24 hours and then dehydrated and embedded in glycol methacrylate. Sections (2 μm thick) cut with glass knives were mounted on microscope slides and stained by PAS technique.

The ocular mucus specimens showed four distinct glycoprotein bands (Figs 51 and 52), designated as GP1, GP2, GP3, and GP4, with GP1 migration slowest and GP4 migration fastest. They appeared to have molecular weights in the range of 300,000 to 2,000,000 daltons. However, the molecular weights of the individual mucus glycoproteins could not be determined accurately because the 200,000-dalton subunit of myosin was the highest molecular weight standard available for SDS gel electrophoresis (Fig 51). The four glycoprotein bands were observed only when the mucus samples were denatured with a combination of 8 mol/1 urea, 2% SDS, and 5% 2-mercaptoethanol. They were not observed when samples were treated only with SDS and 2-mercaptoethanol or with SDS and other reducing agents such as dithiothreitol or N-acetylcysteine, indicating that 8 mol/1 urea is required for complete solubilization of the mucus samples.

The four glycoprotein bands stained positively with both the PAS technique and alcian blue 8GX staining techniques (Fig 51). Coomassie brilliant blue staining of these gels demonstrated only one additional nonglycoprotein band with a molecular weight of approximately 90,000 daltons.

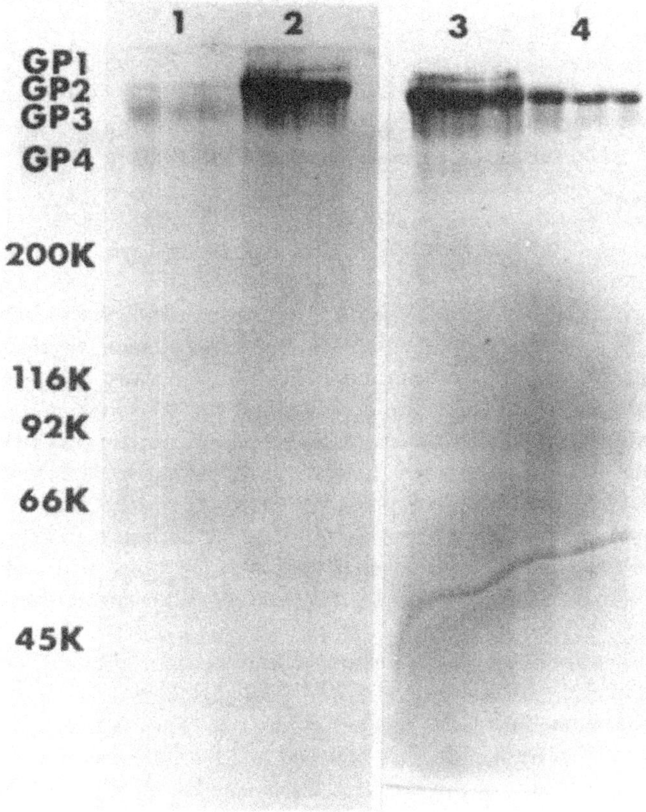

FIGURE 51: Comparison of two ocular mucus samples stained with PAS (lanes 1 and 2) and alcian blue 8GX (lanes 3 and 4) alter electrophoresis on 2% to 16% gradient polyacrylamide gels. Lanes 2 and 3 contained ocular mucus from a patient with atopic conjunctivitis, lanes 1 and 4 contained ocular mucus from a normal individual. Markers to left of gels indicate positions of molecular weight standards: myosin, 200K; β-galactosidase, II6K; phosphorylase A, 92K; bovine serum albumin, 66K; ovalbumin , 45K. GPI = glycoprotein 1, GP2 = glycoprotein 2, GP3 = glycoprotein 3, and GP4 = glycoprotein 4.

Ocular mucus samples from different individuals with normal or inflamed eyes differed slightly in their glycoprotein composition. GP2 was consistently present; GP1, GP3, and GP4, however, were present in some samples and absent in others. Table XVIII shows the frequencies at which different glycoproteins occurred in patients with ocular inflammation.

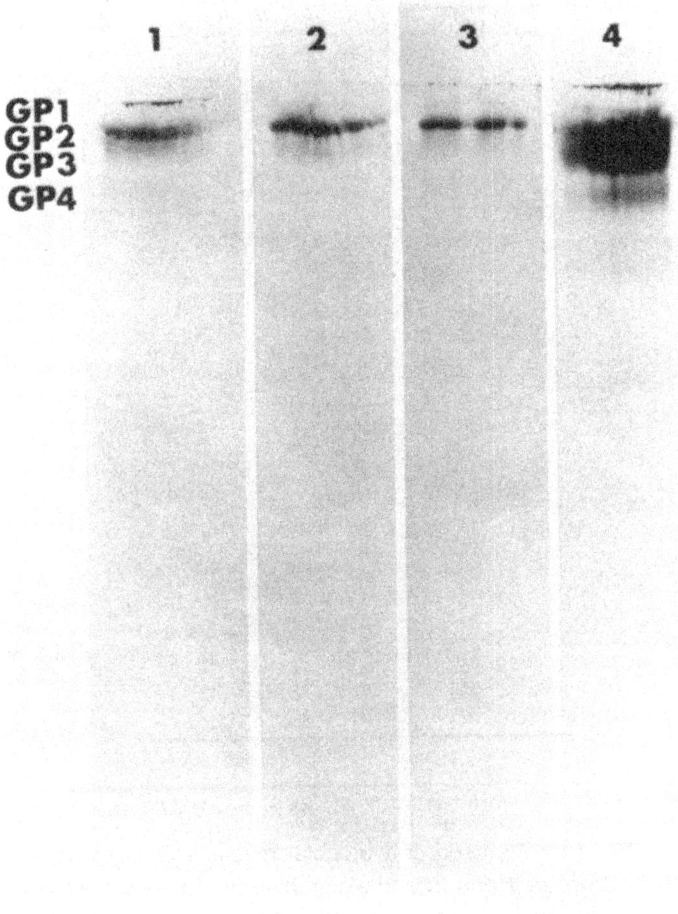

FIGURE 52: Comparison of normal ocular mucus with mucus samples from patients with various types of ocular inflammation. Lane 1, pooled ocular mucus from a normal individual. Lane 2, ocular mucus from a patient with blepharitis. Lane 3, ocular mucus from a patient with Sjogren's disease (keratoconjunctivitis sicca). Lane 4, ocular mucus from a patient with inflammation following extracapsular cataract extraction (2 days postoperatively) (PAS staining). Major mucin glycoproteins are labeled GPI through GP4.

TABLE XVII

CASE	HLA PHENOTYPE
1	A2, BW35, CW4
2	A2, B12
3	A1, A3, B7
4	A3, BW35
5	A2, A3, B27
6	A2, A3, B7
7	A1, A10, BW16
8	A28, BW40
9	A1, A3, B8
10	A9, B21
11	A2, B10, B12
12	A2, A3, B7
13	A3, B27
14	A7, B21
15	A2, A3, B7
16	AW19, B7
17	A11, B5
18	A25, B12
19	A2, A3, B15
20	AW19, B40
21	A1, B15
22	AW24, CW6
23	B12, CW3
24	AW19, CW3
26	AW24, BW44
27	B40, CW3
28	AW19, BW44
29	B12, CW6
30	B7, CW2

TABLE XVIII: GLYCOPROTEIN COMPOSITION OF OCULAR MUCUS (DETERMINED WITH PAS-STAINED GELS) FROM PATIENTS WITH DIFFERENT TYPES OF OCULAR INFLAMMATION

DIAGNOSIS	FREQUENCIES OF GLYCOPROTEINS OBSERVED (%)			
	GP1	GP2	GP3	GP4
Other*	3/10 (30)	10/10 (100)	8/10 (80)	6/10 (60)
CP	5/18 (29)	18/18 (100)	13/18 (72)	11/18 (61)
SJS†	0/4 (0)	4/4 (100)	3/4 (75)	1/4 (25)

*Atopic disease, meibomianitis, superior limbal keratoconjunctivitis, and blepharitis. Numbers in parentheses are percentage.
†Stevens-Johnson syndrome.

Ocular mucus from 18 patients with CP contained the same four glycoproteins that were found in normal individuals or patients with generalized ocular inflammation (Fig 53). An analysis of the frequencies at which the glycoproteins were present in the 18 CP patients studied showed that the four mucus glycoproteins were present at the same frequencies in patients with CP as in normal individuals or patients with other types of ocular inflammation (Table XVIII). However, these mucin glycoproteins were not specific to ocular inflammation, since the same glycoproteins were observed in samples collected from normal individuals. Ocular mucus samples collected from four patients with Stevens-Johnson syndrome showed a glycoprotein composition that was not significantly different from the glycoprotein composition of ocular mucus from CP patients or patients with other types of ocular inflammation (Fig 54). Although GPl was absent in the four patients with Stevens-Johnson syndrome and GP4 was present in only one (Table XVIII), it is entirely possible that these glycoproteins would have occurred at the same frequencies seen in other types of ocular inflammation if more Stevens-Johnson patients had been studied.

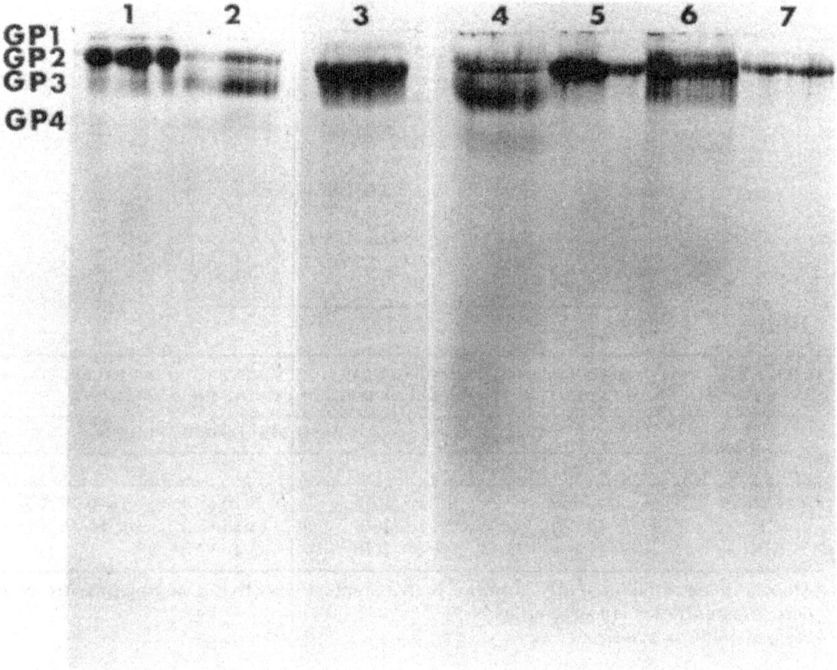

FIGURE 53: Comparison of normal ocular mucus with ocular mucus from patients with ocular CP. Lanes 1 through 6, mucus samples from six patients with CP. Lane 7, pooled ocular mucus from a normal individual (PAS staining). Major mucin glycoproteins are labeled GPI through GP4.

Light microscopic observations of biopsy specimens from patients with CP and Stevens-Johnson syndrome indicated that only one of six

CP patients biopsied and only one of four Stevens-Johnson patients studied possessed goblet cells in limbal conjunctiva. However, all of these patients had normal mucus glycoproteins detectable by gel electrophoresis (Table XIX).

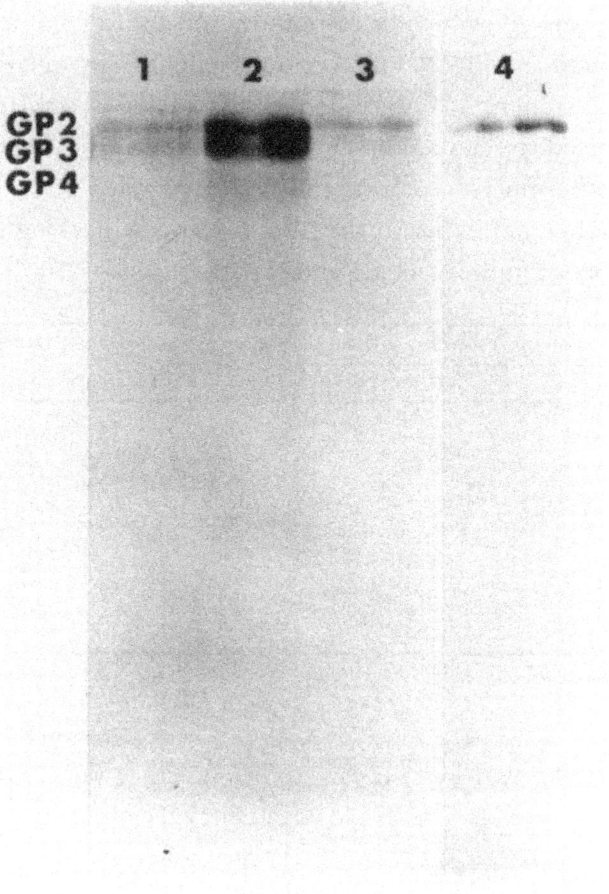

FIGURE 54: Lanes 1 through 4 contain ocular mucus samples from four patients with Stevens-Johnson syndrome (PAS staining). Major mucin glycoproteins are labeled CP2 through CP4.

The techniques described here offer two advantages over previously described analyses of human ocular mucus using SDS-polyacrylamide gel electrophoresis. First, the use of 8 mol/l urea with SDS and 2-mercapto-ethanol causes a more complete dissociation of the mucus polymers into four distinct glycoprotein components. Moore and Tiffany[111] used only SDS and reducing agents, 2-mercaptoethanol, dithiothreitol, or N-acetyl-cysteine, to reduce ocular mucus prior to electrophoresis, while Chao et al[110] utilized SDS and 2-mercaptoethanol. Secondly, the use of 2% to 16% acrylamide gradient separating gels gives greater resolution and more complete separation of the protein and glycoprotein components in the mucus. In previous studies[110,111] straight 15% acrylamide or 5% to 15% acrylamide gradient gels were used to separate mucins glycoproteins. However, due to their large size, the mucus glycoproteins never migrated onto the separating gels, but remained either in the 3% acrylamide stacking gels or at the interface between the stacking and separating gels.

TABLE XIX: COMPARISON OF LIMBAL CONJUNCTIVAL BIOPSY AND GEL ELECTROPHORESIS RESULTS

PATIENT	DIAGNOSIS	GOBLET CELLS*	GP1	GP2	GP3	GP4
1	CP	−	−	+	+	+
2	CP	−	−	+	−	−
3	CP	−	+	+	+	+
4	CP	+	−	+	+	+
5	CP	−	−	+	+	+
6	CP	−	−	+	+	−
7	SJS	−	−	+	−	−
8	SJS	−	−	+	+	+
9	SJS	−	−	+	+	+
10	SJS	−	−	+	+	−

*+, Normal number of goblet cells in limbal conjunctiva; −, no goblet cells observed in limbal conjunctiva.

It is not known from these studies whether GP1, GP2, GP3, and GP4, as observed on 2% to 16% gradient gels, are distinct glycoprotein subunits or whether GP1 and GP2 are polymeric forms of GP3 and GP4. Our estimation of the molecular weight of GP4 (270,000 to 300,000 daltons) is in close agreement with that of Moore and Tiffany[111] for a subunit of ocular mucus, GP3M, with a molecular weight of approximately 200,000 daltons; our GP4 glycoprotein observed on 2% to 16% gradient may be identical to their GP3M subunit. Likewise, GP1 and GP2 described by Moore and Tiffany could be analogous to our GP1, GP2, and GP3, with Moore and Tiffany's GP2 being resolved into two distinct components (GP2 and GP3) on the 2% to 16% gradient gels.

Our finding that limbal conjunctiva from CP and Stevens-Johnson patients had reduced numbers of conjunctival goblet cells despite demonstration of mucin glycoproteins is in agreement with a previous study[102] which demonstrated that patients with CP and radiation keratitis possessed substantial amounts of mucin glycoproteins in their tears despite drastically reduced numbers of conjunctival goblet cells. Dohlman and co-workers[104] have also demonstrated mucus glycoprotein in the tears of patients with CP and Stevens-Johnson syndrome. These and other investigators have pointed out that substantial amounts of mucus glycoproteins might be synthesized and secreted by the lacrimal gland. This notion is supported by histochemical studies that indicate the presence of PAS-positive, alcian blue-positive, neuraminidase-sensitive mucosubstances in the acinar cells of the lacrimal gland. It is also possible that substantial amounts of mucosubstances are produced by the accessory lacrimal gland tissues, since histologic studies have shown these tissues to contain PAS-positive granules.[105] Mucins may also be produced by nongoblet conjunctival epithelial cells in patients with CP and Stevens-Johnson syndrome.[106-108] Although preliminary experiments in our laboratory using a polyclonal antiserum to GP2 indicate that conjunctival goblet cells synthesize this mucin glycoprotein, it may be that the lacrimal gland epithelium also synthesizes GP2. In contrast, Moore and Tiffany[111] demonstrated that antiserum directed against their GP2 reacted only with conjunctival goblet cells and did not react with lacrimal gland tissue.

The mucus harvested from CP and Stevens-Johnson patients in this study consisted primarily of the thick mucus strands in the inferior fornix of these patients. As we suggested above, epithelial cell rupture and lysis during inflammation could contaminate the ocular mucus with cellular protein and intracellular nucleic acids, ribonucleic acid and DNA, causing an increase in the viscosity of mucus. We believe this thickened, contaminated mucus pulls away from the ocular surface and is swept into the inferior fornix by blinking.

It is not known at present whether patients with CP and Stevens-Johnson syndrome possess a functional amount of mucus covering the corneal and conjunctival surfaces. Our preliminary observations with scanning and transmission electron microscopy indicate that mucus is present on the surface of limbal conjunctiva from these patients even though conjunctival goblet cells are not observable in most of these individuals.

Inflammatory Mediators in Tear Film

We suspected that the preocular tear film of patients with CP contained substantial amounts of inflammatory mediators. Preliminary results, reported at ARVO, 1984, confirmed this suspicion, not only for patients with CP but also for individuals with other external inflammatory diseases (rosacea, vernal keratoconjunctivitis, rheumatoid peripheral ulcerative keratitis). In collaboration with Dr. Dwight Robinson, we therefore subjected individual tear samples from patients with CP to high-performance liquid chromatography (HPLC) to determine the presence of arachidonic acid metabolites. Briefly, we employed a Waters Associates, Milford, MA, system for reverse phase HPLC, consisting of an M6000 pump, a model 440 absorbance detector at 280 nm, and a C18 u-Bondpak column. On-line spectrophotometric monitoring at 280 and 220 nm was used as well as other intermediate metabolites according to preestablished standards in our laboratory. Leukotrienes (LTs) were extracted from tears onto Sep-pak C 18 cartridges (Waters) previously rinsed with methanol and water. After applying the tears, we rinsed the columns with water and hexane, elute LTs with methanol. The methanol is removed in a stream of nitrogen and the residue was reconstituted in the HPLC mobile phase. The LT samples were applied and eluted isocratically with a solvent consisting of 67% methanol, 33% water, and 0.08% glacial acetic acid, adjusted to apparent pH 5.5 with 58% aqueous ammonia. One-millimeter fractions were collected at a flow rate of 1 ml/min and prepared for radioimmunoassay by removing the solvent in vacuo with a Speed Vac concentrator (Sanant, Hicksville, NY) and dissolving the residue in Isogel-tris buffer, pH 7.4. Radioimmunoassay of HPLC fractions further established the identity of the HPLC peaks and served as a method of internal validation of LT separation.

Data were subjected to two-way analysis of variance with groups and time as factors.

Tritiated TXB_2 (thromboxane), 6-keto-$PGF_{1\alpha}$., LTB_4, LTC_4, LTD_4, LTE_4, and 5-HETE were from New England Nuclear, Boston, MA. Standards of LTC_4, LTD4, and LTE_4 were generously provided by Dr J. Rokash, Merck-Frosst, Montreal, Canada. Standard TXB_2 and 6-keto-$PGF_{1\alpha}$ was purchased from the Upjohn Co, Kalamazoo, MI. Solvents for HPLC were spectral grade from Burdich and Jackson.

The data from eight CP patients' tears are shown in Table XX.

All the values are highly significant, given that we cannot detect any of these mediators in tears from normal individuals. We suspect that these mediators are toxic to corneal and conjunctival epithelial membranes; studies currently in progress in our laboratory are designed to investigate this question.

CLINICAL TRIALS

Randomized Double-Masked Clinical Trial Comparing Cyclophosphamide with Prednisone vs Prednisone Alone in the Treatment of Progressive CP Affecting the Eyes

Earlier published studies,[71,72] as well as an uncontrolled study of ours,[2] showed that prednisone was less effective than cytotoxic drugs in treating CP, and that the long-term adverse effects of prednisone were unacceptable. Nonetheless, we believed that it was essential, in a small sample of patients, to directly compare prednisone therapy with cyclophosphamide plus prednisone, with respect to the drugs' efficacy and safety. We studied 24 patients with bilateral, stage III CP affecting the eyes. All patients were treated and monitored directly by us. The diagnosis in all cases was based on clinical findings plus a positive biopsy showing, by IF, deposition of at least one immunoreactant at the epithelial BMZ. All patients exhibited stage III conjunctival changes for pemphigoid and were judged, after elimination of potential confounding variables (trichiasis, distichiasis, lagophthalmos, etc) to have active disease, with conjunctival vascular dilatation and infiltration of the substantia propria. Patients with a history of chronic ocular drug use prior to disease onset were excluded, as were patients with histories

TABLE XX: INFLAMMATORY MEDIATOR IN TEARS OF CP PATIENTS

PATIENT*	MEDIATOR CONCENTRATION IN TEARS (ng/ml)					
	THROMBOXANE	PGE_2	6-KETO-$PGF_{1\alpha}$	S-HETE	LBT_4	LTC_4
1	8	10	67	267	221	368
2	27	28	300	350	248	400
3	18	10	105	345	141	281
4	40	27	280	331	213	345
5	35	25	285	295	207	388
6	14	11	114	348	247	351
7	13	12	85	291	156	295
8	29	26	281	275	253	381
Mean	23	18.625	189.625	312.75	210.75	351.125
SD	± 4.044	± 2.999	± 36.999	± 12.181	± 14.925	± 15.254

*Most inflamed eye measured.
PGE_2 = , 6-keto-$PGF_{1\alpha}$ = , S-HETE = , LBT_4 = , LTC_4 =

compatible with conjunctival scarring secondary to infection, trauma, malignancy, or systemic disease (Stevens-Johnson syndrome, sarcoidosis, Sjogren's syndrome, progressive systemic sclerosis).

No patients were eliminated from the study once it began, and none had contraindications to immunosuppression. All patients agreed to a minimum follow-up period of 1 year. Treatment assignments, developed as a result of assignment from a table of random numbers, incomplete block design, were placed in sequentially numbered sealed envelopes. I was an unmasked observer and performed the randomization of treatment assignments, direct treatment of the patient, drug monitoring, and intervention. Each new patient entered into the study was assigned to the treatment designated on the card in the next assignment envelope in sequence. Dr James Kalpaxis, an Ocular Immunology fellow, was a masked observer who rendered opinions regarding disease activity, quiescence, or progression.

Treatment consisted of either a dextrose placebo plus prednisone or cyclophosphamide plus prednisone. Daily prednisone dosage was 1 mg/ kg for 1 week, 0.75 mg/kg for the following 2 weeks, 0.5 mg/kg for the next 2 weeks, 0.25 mg/kg for the 2 weeks following that, and then 0.5 mg/kg every other day for 4 weeks. Patients assigned to the prednisone treatment group were then further tapered to 0.25 mg/kg every other day for another 3 months unless drug-induced complications or treatment failures were judged (Appendix V).

Cytoxan was given at a daily dosage of 2 mg/kg, in conjunction with the above prednisone regimen. In this group, however, the prednisone taper was continued until prednisone was completely discontinued.

Evaluation parameters in the longitudinal study of these patients included visual acuity, degree of conjunctival inflammation (0 to 4+), integrity of the ocular surface epithelium, rose bengal staining pattern, progression of conjunctival cicatrization, symptoms suggesting drug-induced side effects, and results of hemogram, chemistry, and urinalysis. The criteria for successful treatment were: (1) the abolition of all clinical signs of conjunctival inflammation with the globes rendered white and quiet; and (2) the absence of evidence indicating progression of subepithelial fibrosis/conjunctival cicatrization.

The demographic characteristics and relevant clinical information for the study population are shown in Table XXI.

The degree of disease activity (conjunctival clinical inflammatory signs, (0 to 4+), was comparable between the two treatment groups. Women made up 75% of the patients in the immunosuppressed group and 75% of the prednisone group. The average age was 71.50 in the immunosuppressed group and 70.75 in the present prednisone group. Extraocular sites of involvement were noted in 25% of the prednisone group and 58% of the immunosuppressed. None of the patients in either treatment group had other autoimmune systemic diseases or malignancy.

TABLE XXI: DEMOGRAPHIC AND CLINICAL DATA ON 24 PATIENTS WITH CP RANDOMIZED, DOUBLE-MASKED CLINICAL TRIAL COMPARING PREDNISONE VERSUS PREDNISONE AND CYTOXAN THERAPY

	OCULAR INVOLVEMENT						EXTRAOCULAR INVOLVEMENT	
			DURATION (YR)		VISUAL ACUITY			
CASE	SEX	AGE	OD	OS	OD	OS	SITE (S)	DURATION (YR)
1	M	68	8	6	20/70	20/50	Nose, mouth, throat, rectum	8
2	F	72	8	5	20/200	20/70	Pharynx, vagina	8
3	F	80	2	2	20/70	20/400	—	—
4	F	71	1	1	HM*	20/50	Nose	1
5	F	72	2	2	20/400	20/100	—	—
6	M	68	2	2	20/40	20/40	—	—
7	F	73	2	1	20/200	20/25	Mouth, nose	2
8	F	84	3	1	HM	20/40	Mouth, skin	2
9	M	67	1	1	20/70	20/200	—	—
10	F	75	4	5	20/70	20/400	—	—
11	F	74	3	3	20/70	CF@3ft	Throat, nose mouth	3
12	F	85	3	3	20/80	20/200	—	—
13	F	66	1	1	20/200	20/40	Skin	1
14	F	63	1	2	2:/25	20/40	—	—
15	F	75	5	5	20/70	20/70	Nose, mouth	6
16	M	60	1	1	20/50	20/100	Nose, esophagus	1
17	F	77	9	7	20/200	20/100	—	—
18	F	70	2	2	20/100	20/400	—	—
19	F	80	2	Trauma	20/80	—	—	—
20	M	66	1	3	20/30	20/400	Mouth	2
21	F	62	4	4	20/400	20/100	—	—
22	F	70	7	10	20/30	20/400	—	—
23	F	67	2	2	20/70	20/25	—	—
24	M	62	2	2	20/30	20/25	—	—

*HM = hand motion.

The treatment and clinical course of each patient is summarized in Table XXII, and two representative case reports follow. All 12 of the patients treated with cyclophosphamide responded within 8 weeks of institution of therapy. Clinical evidence of active conjunctival inflammation completely subsided, and the globes appeared white and quiet bilaterally. No evidence of recurrent conjunctival inflammation appeared in this group during prednisone taper and discontinuation, nor did cicatrization of the conjunctiva progress during the 6 months of this trial (or at any time after this 6-month observation period ended). All patients in this treatment group at least maintained the visual acuity present when disease activity was brought under control, and acuity improved in eight patients.

TABLE XXII

CASE	THERAPY	CLINICAL COURSE	VISUAL ACUITY AT END OF STUDY (6 MOS)	
			OD	OS
1	CTX[a] + prednisone	W&Q[b] globes by week 6	20/40	20/25
2	Prednisone	Progression; CTX added at week 12; W&Q globes by week 17	HM	20/70
3	CTX + prednisone	W&Q globes by week 5; OS ECCE & PC IOL[c] in week 20	20/70	20/50
4	CTX + prednisone	End stage disease, OD, at start of treatment; W&Q, OS by week 8	HM	20/50
5	Prednisone	Progression; CTX added at week 12; W&Q globes by week 16; severe OD keratopathy[d]	HM	20/200
6	CTX + prednisone	W&Q globes by week 7	20/40	20/40
7	CTX + prednisone	W&Q globes by week 8; OD ECCE & PC IOL in week 20; OS cataract progression	20/40	20/60
8	CTX + prednisone	W&Q globes by week 4; OD epithelial defect healed	20/80	20/30
9	Prednisone	Progression; CTX added at week 12; W&Q globes at week 18; severe OS keratopathy	20/200	CF@3ft
10	CTX + prednisone	W&Q globes by week 8; ECCE & PC IOL OS in week 20; OD cataract progression	20/200	20/50
11	CTX + prednisone	W&Q globes by week 6; dense OS cataract	20/70	CF@3ft

12	Prednisone	Progression; CTX added at week 12; W&Q globes at week 24; keratopathy and cataract	CF@2ft	CF@4ft
13	CTX + prednisone	W&Q globes by week 5; severe OD keratopathy	20/400	20/40
14	CTX + prednisone	W&Q globes by week 7	20/25	20/40
15	Prednisone	Progression; CTX added at week 12; W&Q globes at week 19; severe OS keratopathy	CF@5ft	20/100
16	Prednisone	W&Q globes by week 10; relapse with prednisone taper; dapsone added at end of study	20/50	20/80
17	Prednisone	Progression; CTX added at week 12; W&Q globes by week 21; severe keratopathy, OU	HM@2ft	CF@2ft
18	Prednisone	W&Q globes by week 9; progression of cataracts	20/200	CF@5ft
19	Prednisone	Progression; corneal perforation, OD in week 7, requiring penetrating keratoplasty; CTX added; W&Q globe by week 12	20/400	—
20	CTX + prednisone	W&Q globes by week 8	20/30	20/100
21	Prednisone	W&Q globes by week 7; progression of cataracts	CF@4ft	20/400
22	CTX + prednisone	W&Q globes by week 3	20/40	20/50
23	Prednisone	W&Q globes by week 8; progression of cataracts	20/80	20/40
24	Prednisone	W&Q globes by week 6; progression of cataracts	20/50	20/30

[a]Cytoxan (cyclophosphamide).
[b]White and quiet.
[c]Extracapsular cataract extraction and posterior chamber lens implantation.
[d]Scarring and neovascularization.

TABLE XXIII: ADVERSE EFFECTS OF TREATMENT WITH CYCLOPHOSPHAMIDE AND WITH PREDNISONE

COMPLICATION	CYCLOPHOSPHAMIDE	PREDNISONE
Alopecia	10/12	0
Severe leukopenia	1/12	0
Anemia	12/12	0
Hematuria	1/12	0
Hypertension	0	3/12
Diabetes mellitus	0	2/12
Osteoporosis	0	2/12
Peptic ulcer disease	0	4/12
Myopathy	0	3/12
Psychosis	0	2/12

Complications encountered in the cytotoxic treatment group are shown in Table XXIII. None of the patients withdrew from systemic immunosuppression because of adverse effects, and none required hospitalization for intervention for any side effect. Patients suffered varying degrees of hair loss, but none needed to wear a wig. This adverse side effect proved to be reversible when the drug was discontinued. Leukopenia was a routine finding in all patients successfully treated with cyclophosphamide. Indeed, we have found significant depression in the white blood cell count to be an absolute requirement for achieving the desired therapeutic effect of cyclophosphamide. The leukopenia was reversible, and drug dosage frequently had to be adjusted to achieve the desired level of leukocyte count (2500/ml^3 to 4000/ml^3). Mild to modest degrees of asymptomatic macrocytic anemia developed in all 12 patients. One patient developed reversible microcystic hematuria discovered on routine urinalysis; an alteration in timing of cyclophosphamide adminitration and increased fluid intake eliminated this potentially serious side effect.

Seven of the patients treated with systemic prednisone exhibited incomplete cessation of conjunctival inflammation and showed evidence of progressive conjunctival cicatrization 3 months into therapy. Cyclophosphamide, 2 mg/kg, was added to their therapeutic regimen. Each of these seven patients responded to this addition, and disease activity was completely controlled within 10 weeks.

Five patients in the prednisone treatment group responded completely within 6 weeks with cessation of all signs of conjunctival inflammation. These five patients continued to receive a prednisone maintenance dose, eventually of 0.25 mg/kg every other day, for the 6-month duration of the study period. No evidence of progressive conjunctival cicatrization was seen in these five patients. When the prednisone was tapered further at the end of 6 months, conjunctival inflammation recurred with clinically evident CP activity seen ocularly in all five patients and extraocularly in three patients. Additional chemotherapeutic agents were added: dapsone was employed in all five cases; three cases failed to respond, and azathioprine was employed, 2 mg/kg; the patients responded with a complete cessation of all inflammatory activity.

Each of the patients in the prednisone treatment group experienced prednisone-induced complications. These complications are shown in Table XXIII.

CASE REPORTS

CASE 20

This 66-year-old black man was referred from Pennsylvania in June 1981. In 1978 he had developed the insidious onset of "conjunctivitis" left eye (OS), which gradually worsened until keratopathy developed in the form of epithelial erosions. Vision at that time was reportedly 20/60, and the disease was treated with a variety of topical lubricants, antibiotics, and corticosteroids. In mid 1979 a symblepharon was noted in the OS inferior fornix, and the diagnosis of CP was entertained. Treatment was with lubricants and topical steroids. Symblepharon formation and fornix foreshortening progressed, and subtle changes of subepithelial fibrosis developed in the right eye (OD). Corneal neovascularization developed OS, even though trichiasis, distichiasis, and sicca syndrome were absent (Schirmer evaluation revealed 20 mm of wetting).

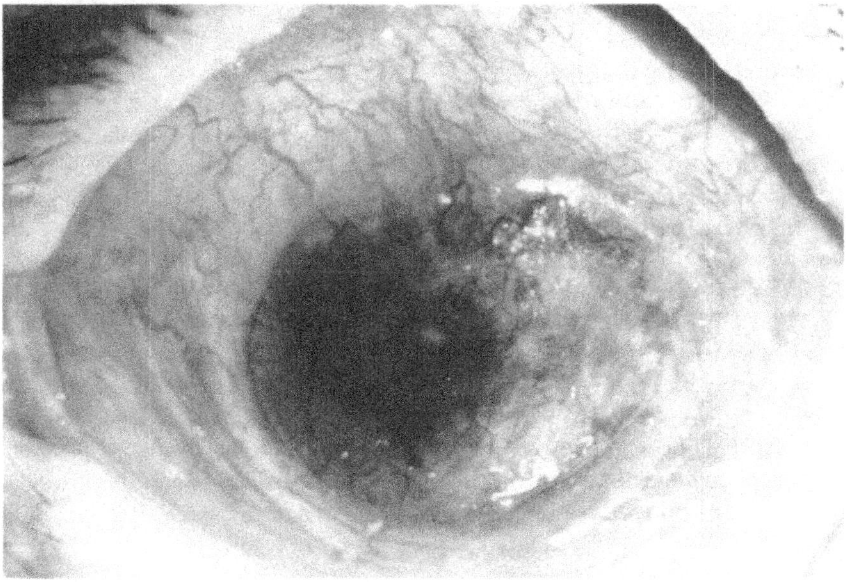

FIGURE 55: Case 20: Left eye, 4+ conjunctival injection, with extreme keratopathy and corneal neovascularization; stage III conjunctival cicatrization.

On our first evaluation of the patient, his visual acuity was 20/30 OD and 20/400 OS. Slit lamp biomicroscopy revealed what appeared to be stage II CP changes OD, with subepithelial fibrosis and fornix foreshortening, and stage III pemphigoid OS, with extensive symblepharon and extreme degrees of keratopathy with corneal neo-vascularization and epithelial erosions (Fig 55). Conjunctival biopsy confirmed the suspicion of CP with IgA and IgG deposition at the epi-thelial BMZ. Subclinical lesions were also detected in the buccal muco-sa and pharynx. Treatment was with oral prednisone, 100 mg/day, an oral cyclophosphamide, 175 mg/day. By 8 weeks into therapy the conjunctival inflammatory response had receded, and by 12 weeks into therapy, visual acuity had improved to 20/100 (Fig 56). The disease remained quiescent throughout the treatment period, and the patient was off all prednisone 10 weeks after the institution of therapy.

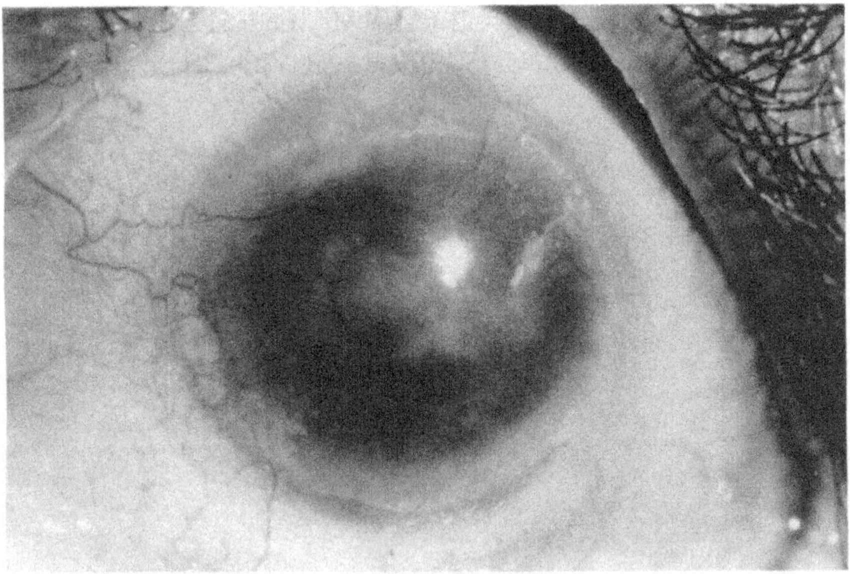

FIGURE 56: Same eye as in Fig 55, 12 weeks after institution of systemic cyclophosphamide therapy.

CASE 15

A 75-year-old woman was first referred to us in August 1980, for evaluation of a chronic conjunctivitis and history of persistent epithelial defects in both eyes (OU). Visual acuity was 20/400 OU. Intraocular pressures were normal. Stromal cellular infiltration, 4+ conjunctival injection, and trichiasis of the lower lids were seen OU, and marked subepithelial fibrosis, fornix foreshortening, and symblepharon formation were noted (Fig 57). Slit lamp biomicroscopy revealed bilateral central corneal epithelial defects and corneal neovascularization. The rest of the examination was unremarkable, with Schirmer testing revealing 13 mm of wetting OU, after topical anesthetic. This patient, in our randomized study, was assigned to the prednisone treatment group. The conjunctival inflammation resolved and the epithelial defects healed with bandage soft lens, topical lubrication, and 1% prednisone acetate drops given four times daily. Conjunctival inflammation recurred on prednisone taper; further corneal damage developed during the subsequent 8 weeks required for successful immunosuppression and control of the inflammation. The final visual acuities were counting fingers (CF) at 5 ft OD, and 20/100 OS (Fig 58).

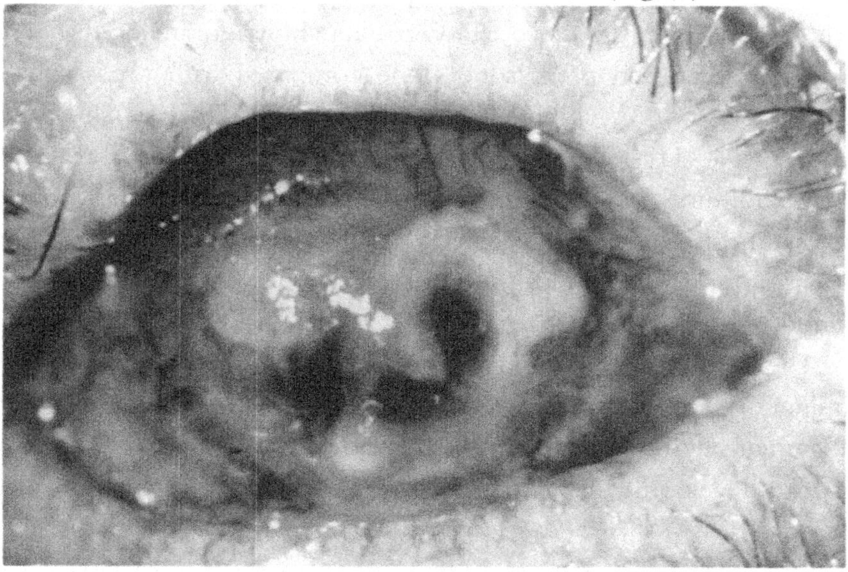

FIGURE 57: Case 15: 4+ conjunctival injection, corneal neovascularization, epithelial defect, and white blood cell infiltration of corneal stroma. Stage III cicatrization of conjunctiva.

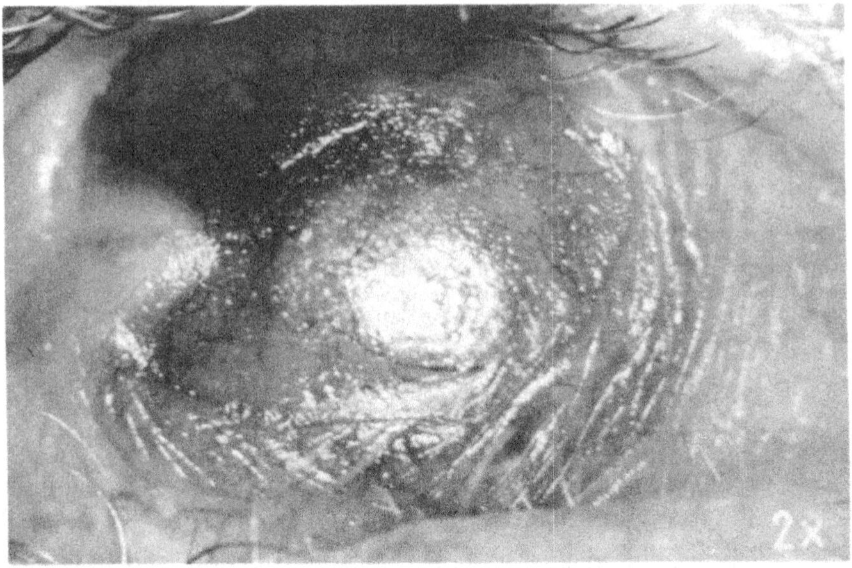

FIGURE 58: End stage disease, stage IV, with epidermalization of ocular surface.

The results of this double-masked, randomized, controlled clinical trial confirms the accuracy of clinical impressions based on previous uncontrolled trials[1,2,71,72] of the therapeutic efficacy of immunosuppressive therapy for progressive CP. Our data show a dramatic difference in efficacy between prednisone alone compared with prednisone in combination with cyclophosphamide. Chi-square analysis shows this difference is statistically significant ($P < 0.005$). Figs 59 through 64 show additional before and after cyclophosphamide therapy photographs in this series. Figs 65 through 68 show an additional case treated with prednisone, topical retinoids, and topical and subconjunctival steroids.

The histopathologic and immunopathologic abnormalities in CP conjunctiva are, in large measure, reversible with control of the chronic inflammation through systemic chemotherapy *if* control is achieved prior to development of extreme (stage IV) permanent structural alterations.

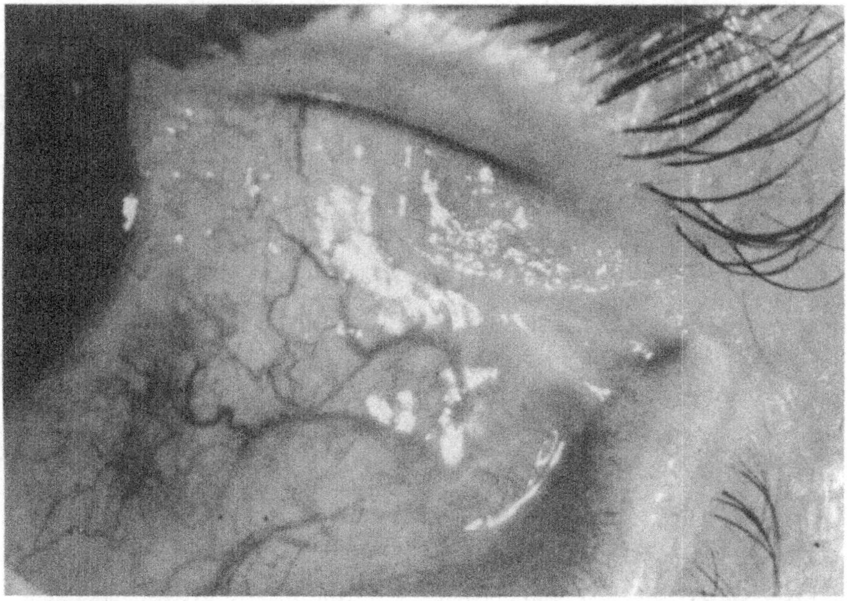

FIGURE 59: Left eye, stage III pemphigoid, prior to institution of cyclophosphamide therapy

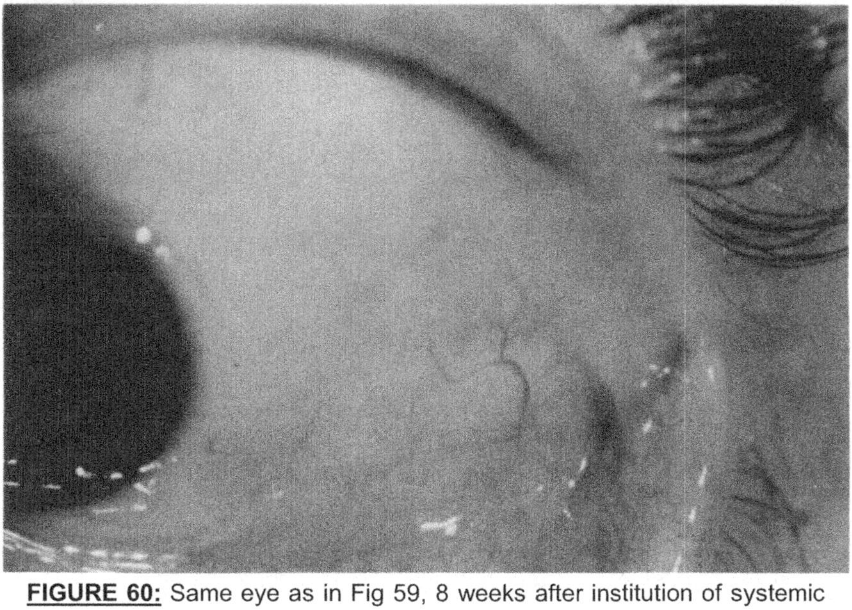

FIGURE 60: Same eye as in Fig 59, 8 weeks after institution of systemic cyclophosphamide therapy.

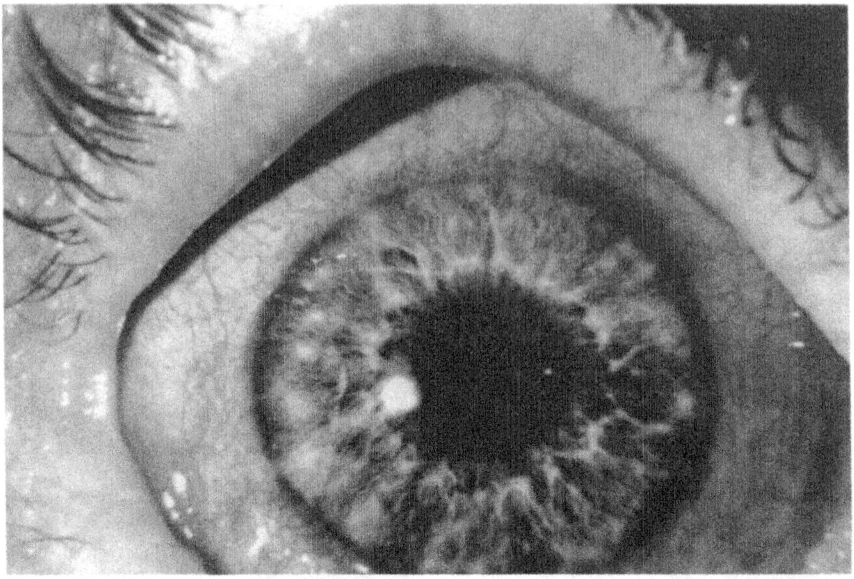

FIGURE 61: Stage III pemphigoid, right eye, prior to cyclophosphamide therapy.

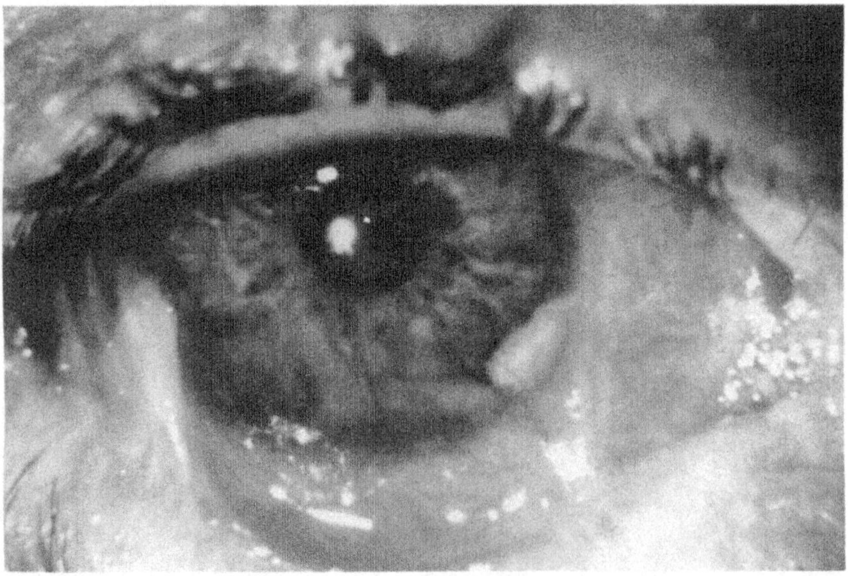

FIGURE 62: Left eye of same patient in Fig 61, prior to therapy.

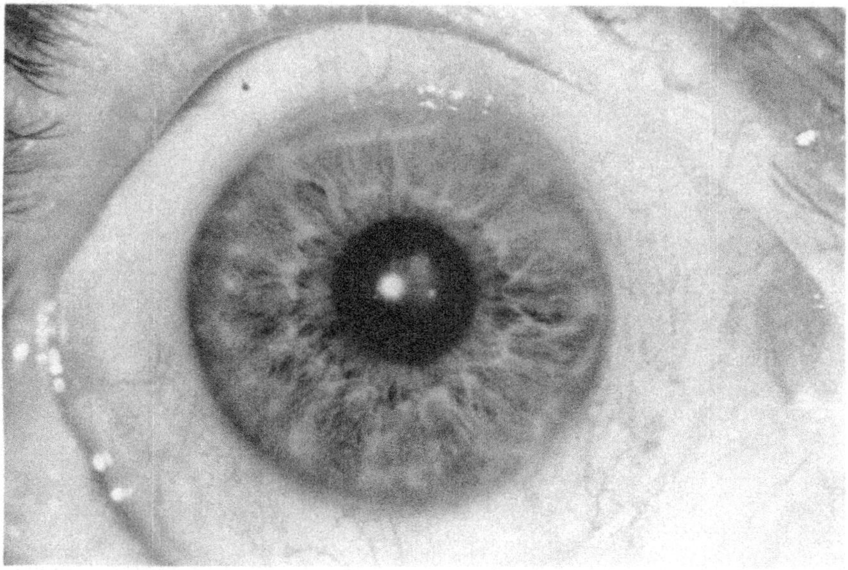

FIGURE 63: Right eye, same patient as in Fig 61, 16 weeks into treatment with systemic cyclophosphamide.

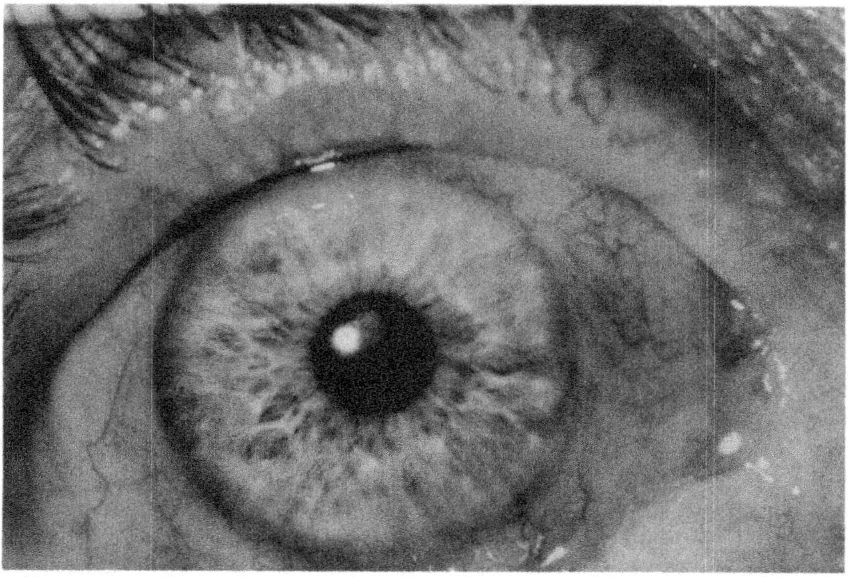

FIGURE 64: Left eye, same patient as in Fig 62, 16 weeks into therapy with systemic cyclophosphamide.

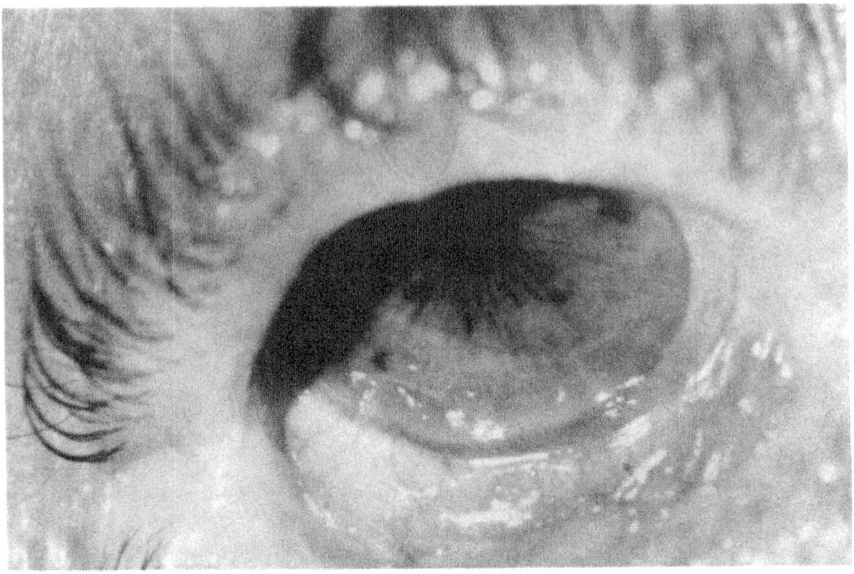

FIGURE 65: Right eye, stage III pemphigoid treated, over an 18-month period, with topical retinoids, systemic prednisone, and topical and subconjunctival prednisone.

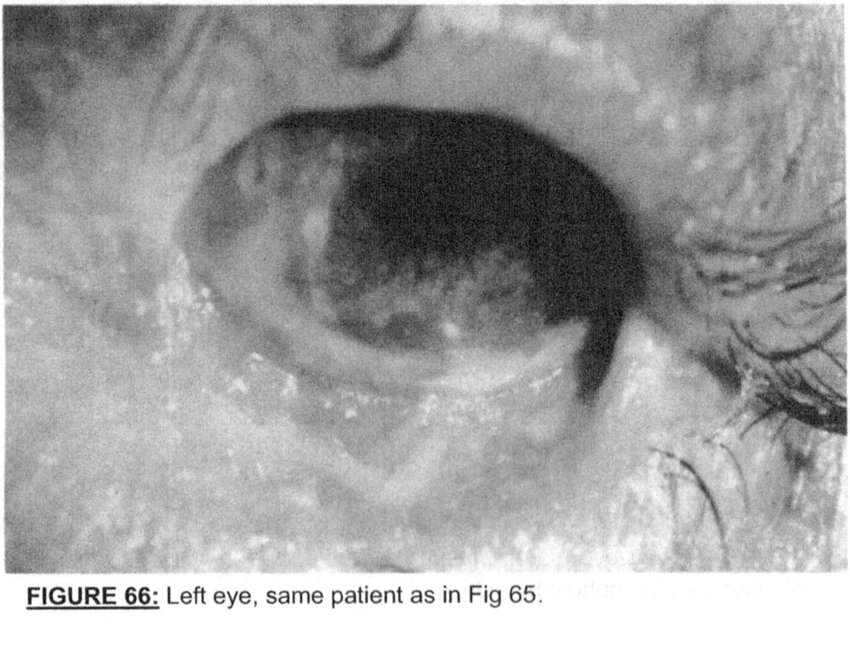

FIGURE 66: Left eye, same patient as in Fig 65.

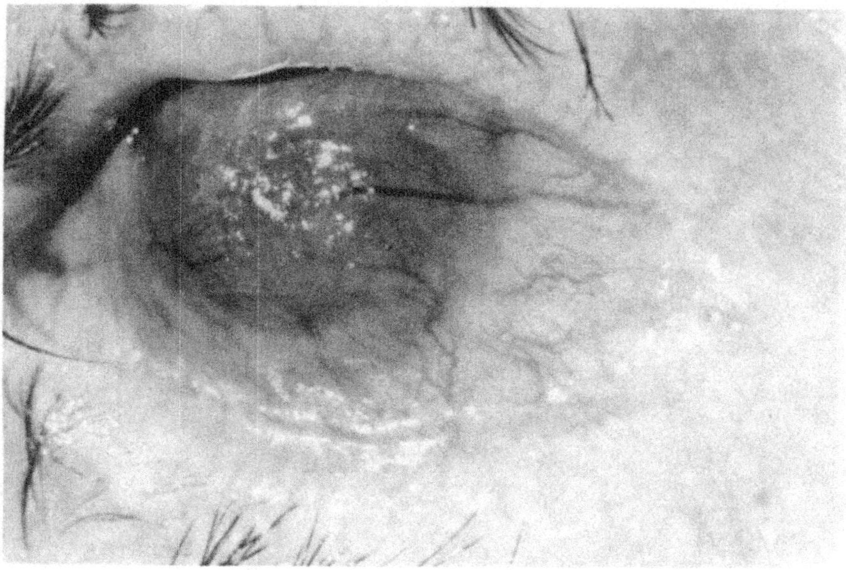

FIGURE 67: Right eye, same patient as in Fig 65, 18 months after the photograph in Fig 65 was taken. Note progressive conjunctival cicatrization and keratopathy.

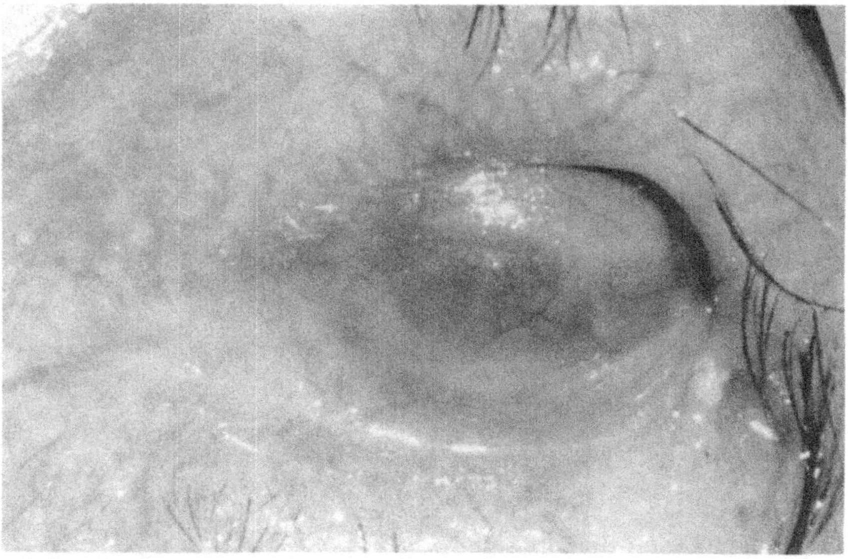

FIGURE 68: Left eye, same patient as in Fig 66, after 18-months therapy with steroids and retinoids. Stage IV conjunctival changes are now present, with ankyloblepharon formation and keratinization of ocular surface.

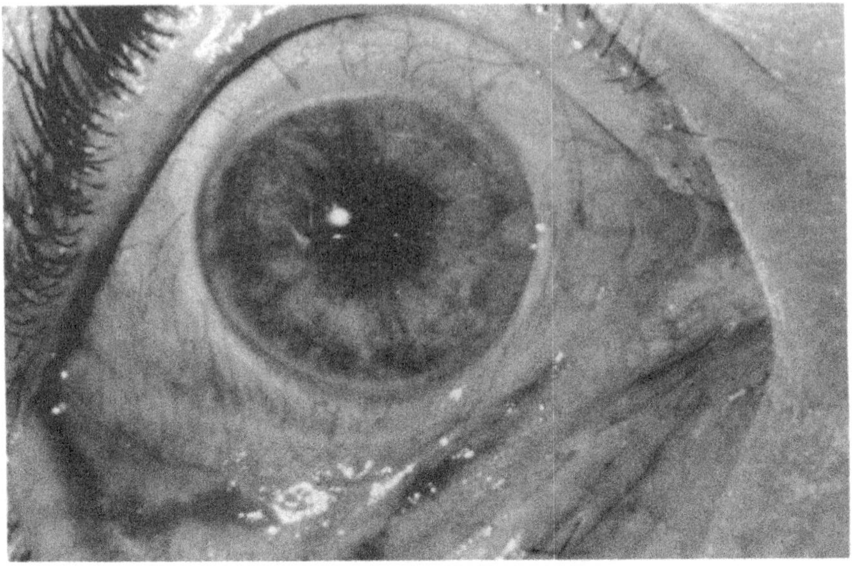

FIGURE 69: OD stage III active CP.

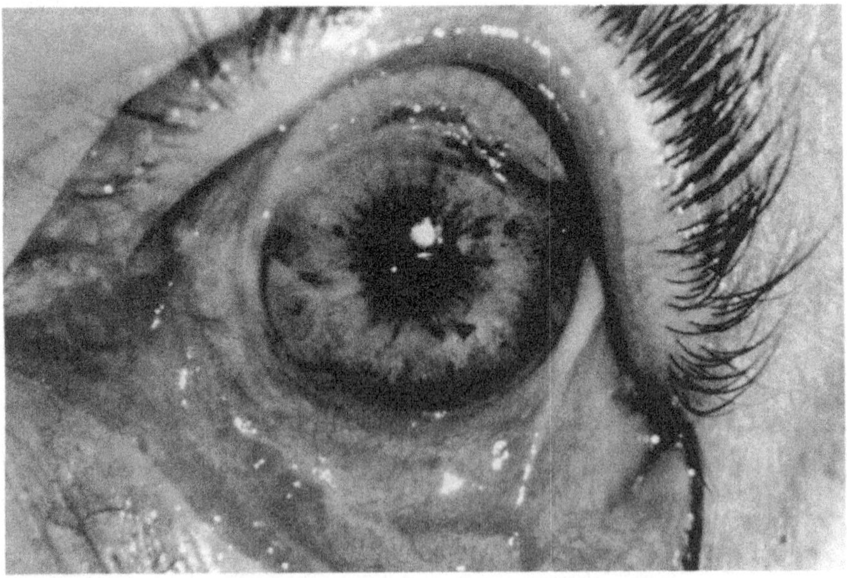

FIGURE 70: OS stage III active CP, same patient as in Fig 69.

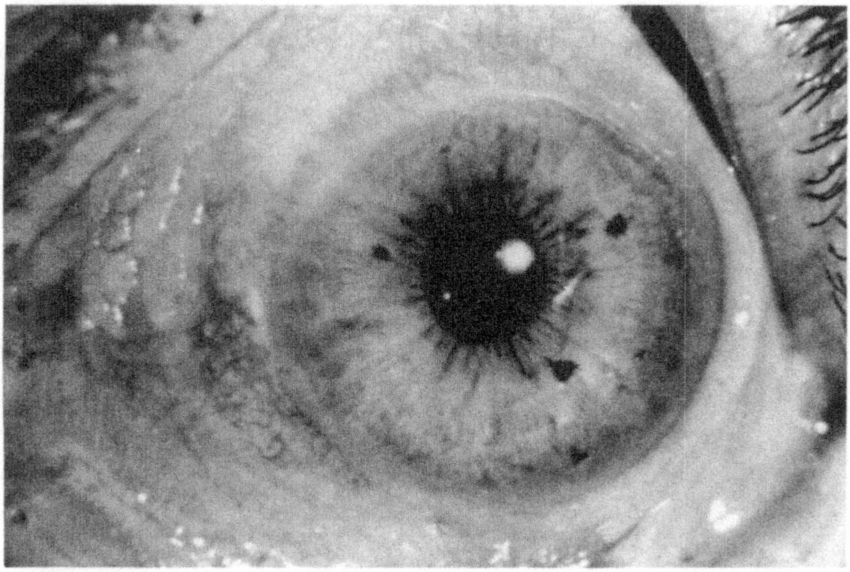

FIGURE 71: Left eye, same patient as in Fig 70. Note large, vertically crescent-shaped patch of keratinized bulbar conjunctival epithelium on nasal aspect of globe.

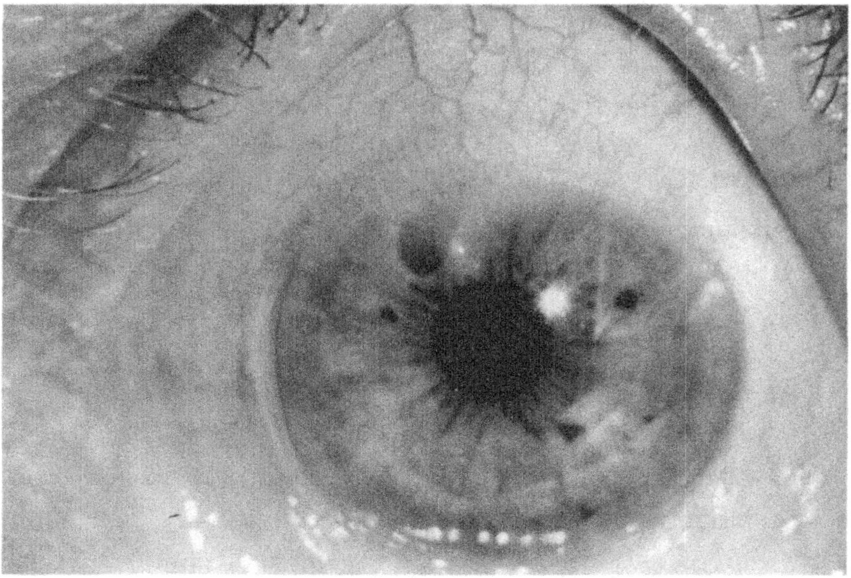

FIGURE 72: Same eye as in Fig 71, after successful control of disease activity with cyclophosphamide. Note disappearance of keratinized epithelium from bulbar conjunctiva.

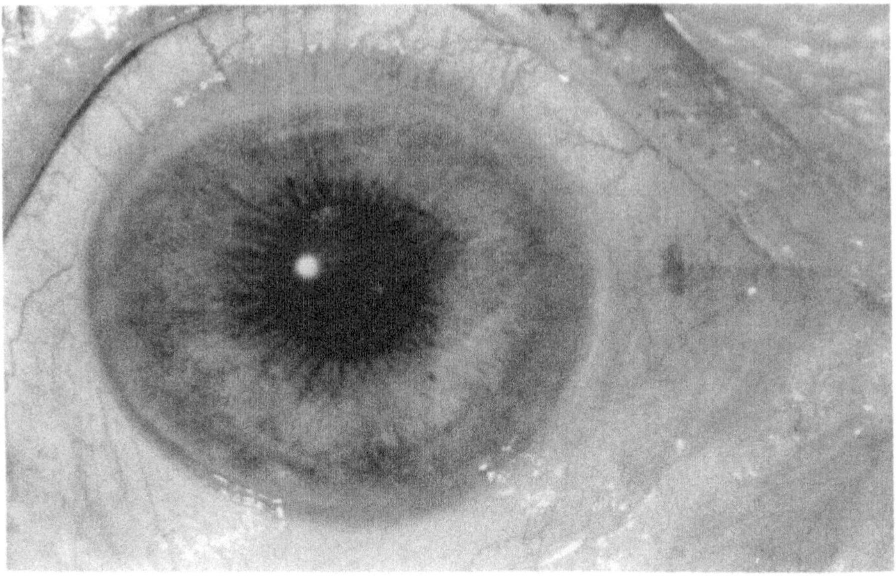

FIGURE 73: Right eye, same patient as in Fig 72, after control of disease activity.

Figs 69 through 72 show that clinically obvious reversal of some pathologic features is also typical of successful control of inflammation. The patient in these photographs exhibits stage III conjunctival cicatrization bilaterally (Figs 69 and 70). The large patch of keratinized bulbar conjunctival epithelium (nasal aspect, OS, Fig 71) gradually reverts to nonkeratinized epithelium (Fig 72) with 6 months of control of the inflammatory activity with cyclophosphamide.

Several points regarding this clinical trial deserve emphasis. First, we treated only patients with unequivocal CP with active, bilateral conjunctival inflammation and progressive conjunctival cicatrization. Second, we treated all factors which could contribute to conjunctival inflammation (sicca, trichiasis, exposure, meibomianitis), in order to eliminate confusion regarding immunologically-driven inflammatory activity. Third, once ocular involvement in CP has reached stage III, further progression and loss of vision due to corneal damage can occur with astonishing rapidity; our results in cases 2, 5, 9, 12, 15, 17, and 19, treated with prednisone, emphasize this point and confirms the similar observation previously published by Mondino and Brown.[22] Fourth, even in those cases treated successfully with prednisone, relapse with prednisone taper occurred routinely; maintenance of prednisone doses sufficient to control CP activity was associated with an extraordinary rate of drug-induced morbidity, including cataract enhancement (cases 9, 12, 15, 18, 21, and 23).

We believe that the results of this study show that systemic immunosuppression is effective in the treatment of CP, and that such therapy, when used properly, poses fewer risks than does long-term corticosteroid therapy. These ideas are not new in the dermatologic literature[68-75] but they are relatively novel for ophthalmologists, so this approach may be considered excessively aggressive by some.

Our therapeutic guidelines are similar to those of many rheumatologists who use systemic immunosuppression for Wegener's granulomatosis, polyarteritis nodosa, systemic lupus erythematosus, or severe rheumatoid arthritis. We offer systemic immunosuppressive therapy only to those patients with progressive disease; we do not treat those with quiescent or endstage disease. The patients are carefully educated about the possible risks and benefits of therapy, and about diagnostic procedures and longitudinal follow-up care. Sperm banking is done for men who wish it, and a careful review of systems for evaluating systemic disease or extraocular sites of involvement is performed. Patients who choose to enter therapy must be followed up longitudinally by a physician experienced in the use of immunosuppressive agents, in proper surveying for therapeutic dose and side effects, and in the management of complications, should they occur.

The complication rate in this series was less than that usually seen in series involving cancer patients. This is probably because the dosages of cytotoxic drugs employed in our series were considerably lower than those required to treat malignancy. It is important, however, to remain vigilant, especially for the potentially lethal complications such as severe bone marrow depression, infection, hemorrhagic cystitis, hemorrhagic colitis, toxic hepatitis, and interstitial pulmonary fibrosis.

Finally, although no causal relationship between cytotoxic therapy and development of neoplasms has been established, especially in patients who do not already have a malignancy, we believe that patients considering systemic immunosuppression should be aware that such a relationship may exist.

Randomized Double-Masked Cliniical Trial Comparing Dapsone with Cyclophosphamide in the Treatment of Progressive CP Affecting the Eyes

Person and Rogers[74] reported that dapsone was effective in the treatment of bullous pemphigoid, and Rogers and associates[75] reported similar efficacy of this drug in the treatment of CP in 24 patients, 17 of whom had ocular involvement. Eighty-three percent of the patients had partial or complete control, with little or no residual inflammatory activity. Twelve of the 17 patients with ocular involvement responded (70%), 5 completely and 7 partially.

We studied 40 patients with active, progressive stage III CP affecting the conjunctiva, employing a study protocol identical to the one described in the preceding section. Briefly, patients were randomized, by envelope opening, into either dapsone or cyclophosphamide treatment groups. The treatment assignment cards were generated, by a computer random number generator, for an incomplete block design, sealed in sequentially numbered envelopes, and were opened in sequence by me in the presence of another observer as each new patient was admitted to the study. The admission and exclusion criteria for the study were as described above, with the additional requirement that the glucose-6-phosphate dehydrogenase screening test result was within normal limits.

The dose of dapsone employed was 2 mg/kg. The dose of cyclophosphamide was 2 mg/kg. Patients were monitored weekly for 1 month, then every 2 weeks thereafter, as described above. Masked observer determinations of conjunctival inflammatory activity and cicatrization progression were also as described above.

The clinical data on the 40 patients in this trial are summarized, for the sake of space economy, in Table XXIV.

The demographic and clinical characteristics were relatively comparable between the two treatment groups. Two women in the dapsone group had rheumatoid arthritis and moderately severe sicca syndrome; one woman in the cyclophosphamide group had this associated disorder. Some of the patients had acne rosacea. Again, in the interest of space, we will report here a narrative summary of the treatment and clinical course of these two treatment groups.

All 20 of the cyclophosphamide therapy patients responded to treatment with an abolition of all clinical evidence of conjunctival inflammation and no evidence of conjunctival scarring throughout the 6-month observation period or beyond. Fourteen of the 20 dapsone-treated patients (70%) responded to treatment. Four patients responded incompletely to dapsone, with reduced but not abolished inflammation, and two patients failed to respond at all within 12 weeks, even at maximal (200 mg/day) doses of dapsone. These six patients were treated with cyclophosphamide after dapsone was discontinued; all responded promptly (within 8 weeks) to this treatment.

TABLE XXIV: SUMMARY OF CLINICAL CHARACTERISTICS OF 40 PATIENTS WITH ACTIVE, PROGRESSIVE STAGE III CP

	DAPSONE (20)	CYCLOPHOSPHAMIDE (20)
Average age	62.4	67.1
Females	15	12
Extraocular sites	8	11
Conjunctival inflammation		
1+	0	0
2+	4	0
3+	12	14
4+	4	6

TABLE XXV: COMPLICATIONS ASSOCIATED WITH DAPSONE IN 20 CP PATIENTS

	ANEMIA	NAUSEA	HEPATITIS	ABDOMINAL PAIN	NEUROPATHY
No. of cases	19	4	1	2	1

The side effects observed in the patients receiving cyclophosphamide included alopecia, anemia and leukopenia, as expected. Two patients developed microcystic hematuria which necessitated a reduction in cyclophosphamide dosage.

The side effects observed in the patients receiving dapsone are shown in Table XXV. It should bc emphasized that dapsone is not a benign drug. Deaths associated with dapsone use have occurred as a result of agranulocytosis, aplastic anemia, and hemolytic anemia.

We found evidence of hemolysis in 19 of our 20 patients on this drug, in spite of the fact that none was glucose-6-phosphate dehydrogenase deficient. These patients experienced a fall in hemoglobin of 1.0 to 3.4 gm/dl, and all showed reticulocytosis (3% to 9%). Nausea, vomiting, and episodic abdominal discomfort occurred in seven patients. Peripheral neuropathy developed in one patient while on 200 mg of dapsone/day; this defect subsided when the drug was stopped.

Dapsone is a sulfone derivative (4-4' diaminodiphenylsulfone) used primarily to treat leprosy. It was found to be effective in the treatment of dermatitis herpetiformis and bullous pemphigoid,[74] and in some patients with CP.[75] Our results confirm these impressions from uncontrolled studies.

The mechanism of action of dapsone may relate to its inhibition of peroxide systems in several types of inflammatory cells; this is speculative, however, and definition of the cellular and molecular events responsible for the antiinflammatory effect of dapsone in CP patients awaits further study.

The six dapsone treatment failures included all four of the patients with 4+ conjunctival inflammation prior to therapy; the two remaining treatment failures had 3+ activity before treatment. If one considers only those patients with mild-to-modest inflammatory activity, 14 of 16 (88%) responded to dapsone. This suggests that dapsone is a reasonable first time drug of choice for cases of CP which are not extremely active and rapidly progressive, provided the patient is not glucose-6-phosphate dehydrogenase-deficient. If dapsone is effective in a CP patient it will produce a reduction in conjunctival inflammation within 4 weeks (Figs 74 and 75). We now usually begin treatment with 25 mg twice daily for 1 week, observing for drug tolerance and for hemolysis. We usually increase the dose to 50 mg twice daily and make additional dosage adjustments based on therapeutic response and on drug tolerance.

Other Immunosuppressive Agents

One hundred eight of the 130 patients in our study population have been treated with dapsone and/or with an immunosuppressive agent. The remaining 12 patients were unwilling to use these drugs; they were treated with corticosteroids, in varying dosages and routes of administration. All of these patients received oral prednisone and topical prednisoone acetate; most also receive subconjunctival injections of betamethasone. Conjunctival cicatrization has progressed in each of these 12 patients during the 2 to 9 years of follow-up, and keratopathy progression has produced profound loss of vision in each.

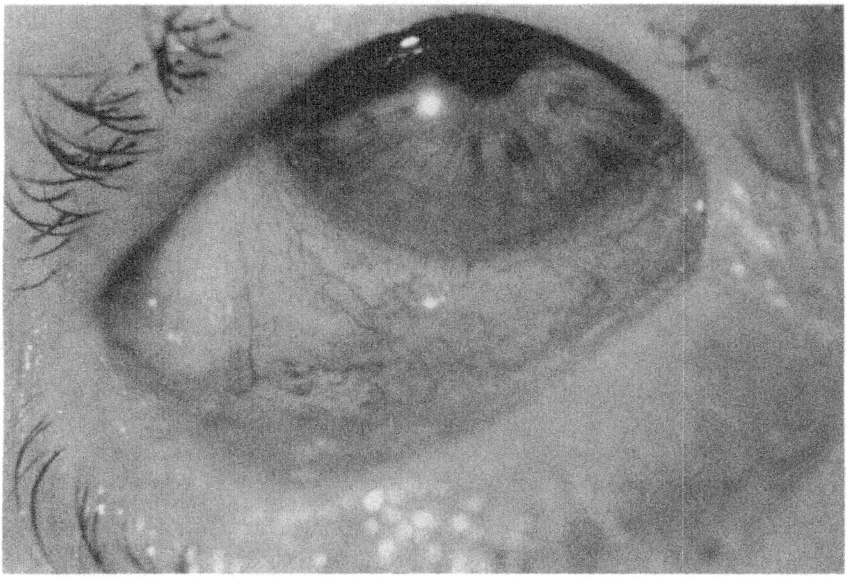

FIGURE 74: Stage III pemphigoid, 2+ inferior fornix inflammatory activity.

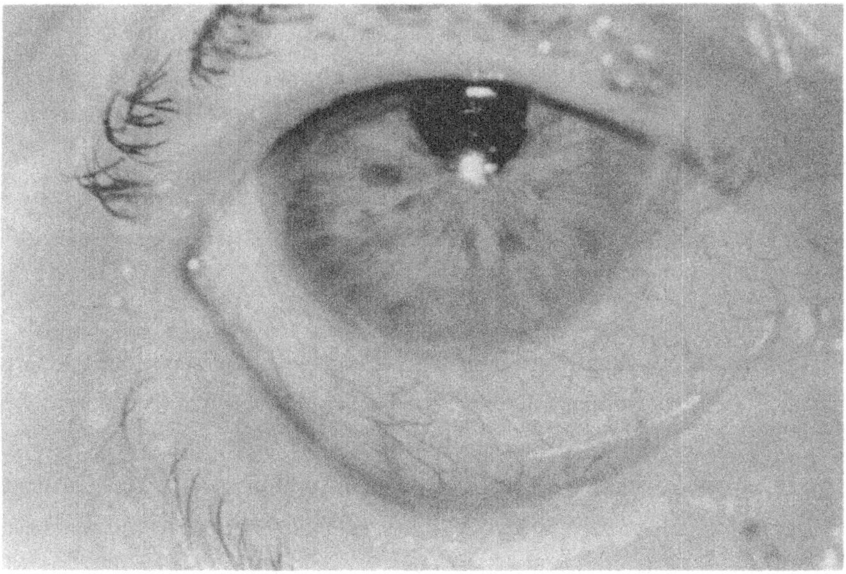

FIGURE 75: Same patient as in Fig 74, 12 weeks after institution of systemic dapsone therapy, with resultant resolution of inflammatory therapy.

Azathioprine, methotrexate and cyclosporine have been employed in the care of selected patients intolerant to cyclophosphamide or dapsone, or therapeutically unresponsive to dapsone. A series of seven patients were treated with oral cyclosporine, 10 mg/kg as initial therapy; all but one of these patients failed to respond adequately to therapy. The one treatment success with cyclosporine is a unique case.

CASE REPORT

This 46-year-old white woman developed bilateral chronic conjunctivitis in the summer of 1979. Her past medical history was remarkable for a Coomb's positive hemolytic anemia, diagnosed in 1969, pernicious anemia, and autoimmune neutropenia. She had had a splenectomy in 1970, and had been on varying doses of oral prednisone since that time. The patient had diabetes mellitus treated with insulin since 1975. The patient has a history of oral and vaginal mucosa ulcers, arthritis, and erythema nodosum, and therefore was diagnosed as having Behçet's syndrome.

At the time of our first evaluation of her she had bilateral conjunctival subepithelial fibrosis, with fornix foreshortening, symblepharon, trichiasis, and distichiasis. IF of a conjunctival biopsy specimen showed C_3, C_4, and IgA deposition at the epithelial BMZ.

The white blood count showed 3000 cells/mm^2, with 40% neutrophils, 55% lymphocytes, and 5% monocytes. The RF was positive (79 IU/ml), the hemolytic complement was depressed to 100 U (normal range, 150 to 250 U), C_3 and C_4 components of complement in the serum were depressed to 73 and 12 mg/dl, respectively (normal values, 83 to 177 mg/dl for C_3 and 15 to 45 mg/dl for C_4), and the ANA was positive, homogeneous pattern, at a titer of 1:32.

Vision OD was 20/40 (Fig 76); a neovascularized cornea with a central epithelial defect and shallow stromal ulcer was present in the left cornea, and the vision in the OS was CF at 2 ft (Fig 77).

Cryoablation of the trichitic lashes, punctal occlusion, OS, for sicca syndrome, and institution of dapsone, 25 mg three times a day, resulted in improvement in vision to 20/25 OD, and 20/200 OS; conjunctival inflammatory activity decreased from 3+ to 1+ OD, and

4+ to 2+ OS. The dapsone dose was eventually escalated to 50 mg three times a day. Variable degrees of neutropenia were attributed to the dapsone use and therefore this drug was discontinued. Conjunctival inflammatory activity relapsed to 2+ OD and 3½+ OS. Cyclophosphamide, 50 mg/day, was begun on June 16, 1983. Neutropenia necessitated withdrawal of that drug. On September 22, 1983, 25 mg of azathioprine was begun. This drug was discontinued on November 3, 1983 because of neutropenia. Prednisone was increased to 40 mg/day; after the patient had been on this dose of prednisone for 3 months, the conjunctival inflammatory activity was 3+ OD, and 4+ OS; visual acuity had fallen to hand movements at 3 ft, OS. Vincristine, 2 mg once a week intravenously was begun. Progressive conjunctival cicatrization over the next 4 weeks necessitated discontinuation of vincristine.

Cyclosporine, 300 mg/day was begun on March 1, 1984. By March 22, 1984, conjunctival inflammatory activity had fallen to 2+ OU, and the white blood count had climbed from 1900 to 8900, with 59% neutrophils.

At the time of the patient's last evaluation in December 1985, visual acuity was 20/25 OD (Fig 78), and CF at 4ft OS (Fig 79). Conjunctival inflammatory activity was judged to be ½+ OD, and 1+ OS. No progressive fibrosis had been observed since the patient had been on cyclosporine. The prednisone dose had been tapered to 10 mg every other day. The cyclosporine dose was 400 mg/day. The white blood count was 6200, with 71% neutrophils. The hematocrit was 35. No mouth ulcers or joint pains had been experienced in the past year. Renal function has remained normal, with a creatinine clearance of 91 ml/minute and serum blood urea nitrogen of 22.

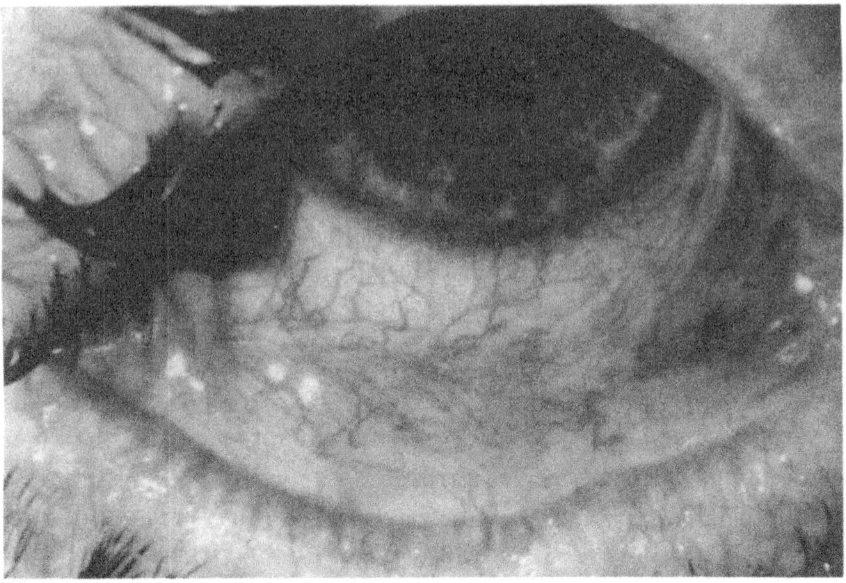

FIGURE 76: Right eye, stage III CP, in a patient with multiple autoimmune phenomenon.

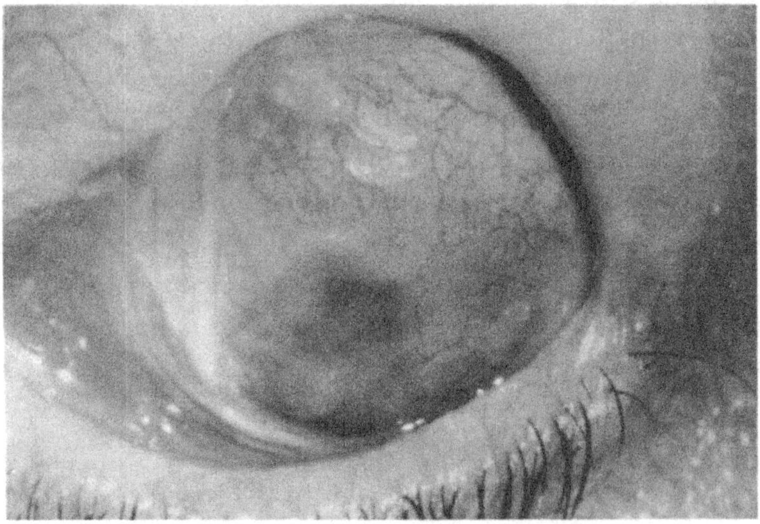

FIGURE 77: Same patient as in Fig 76, left eye, with epithelial defect and corneal neovascularization.

Treatment Failures

Ten of the 118 (8.5%) patients treated with systemic chemotherapeutic regimens have failed to respond adequately; each of these patients experienced progressive conjunctival cicatrization, keratopathy development and progression, and profound visual loss. Analysis of these cases, in an effort to discover some unifying feature, discloses a disproportionate number of males in the group (8 of 10 or 80%), considering that females predominate in the total study population of our CP patients (64%). The two female patients had concommitant rheumatoid arthritis with associated sicca syndrome; these patients developed persistent corneal epithelial defects, secondary microbial keratitis, progressive corneal stromal ulceration, corneal perforation, and endophthalmitis.

The demographic characteristics of the eight males who responded in-completely to treatment are shown in Table XXVI, along with ocular and extraocular manifestations at the time of onset of the disease.

Three remarkable features from the data in Table XXVI are the dramatic asymmetry of ocular involvement in these cases, the fact that all had profound sicca syndrome, and all had extraocular manifestations. None of the patients had an associated autoimmune disease, and none had detectable circulating autoantibodies (ANA, RF, or anti-BMZ antibody). All of the patients exhibited facial skin changes strongly suggestive of acne rosacea: dilated and plugged sebaceous ducts, telangiectasias, extremely oily skin; lid findings in these patients included lid thickening, lid margin telangiectasias, and meibomian duct plugging, with thick meibum expressible with effort.

TABLE XXVI: MALE CP PATIENTS INCOMPLETELY RESPONSIVE TO CHEMOTHERAPY

CASE	AGE AT ONSET	STAGE		VISUAL ACUITY		EXTRAOCULAR MANIFESTATIONS
		OD	OS	OD	OS	
1	54	III	II	CF	20/60	Esophagus, nose
2	69	II	IV	20/70	CF	Mouth, nose, throat
3	74	III	II	20/400	20/400	Nose, skin
4	41	II	IV	20/70	HM	Throat, mouth
5	60	II	III	20/30	20/100	Mouth, esophagus
6	77	IV	III	CF	20/100	Nose, mouth
7	58	II	III	20/50	20/200	Esophagus, mouth
8	63	III	III	20/80	20/400	Mouth, nose

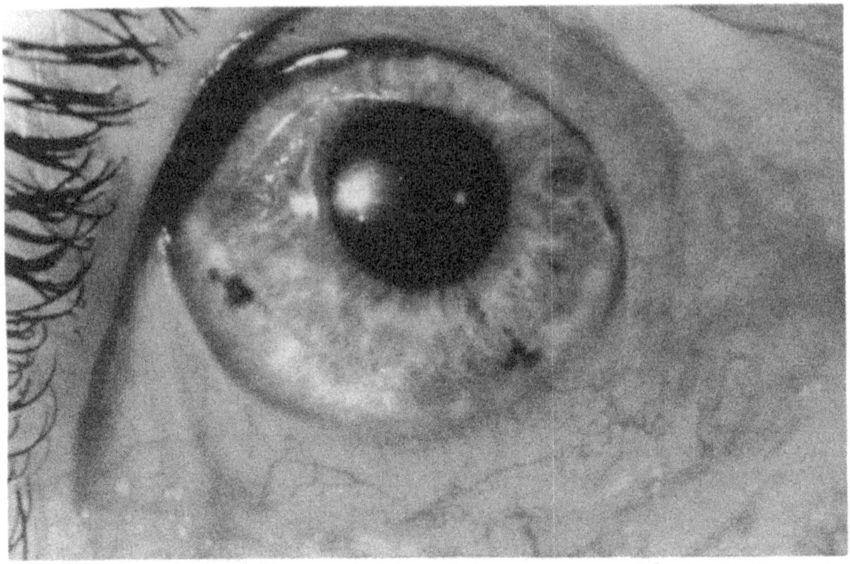

FIGURE 78: Same eye as in Fig 76, 6 weeks after institution of cyclosporine therapy orally. Note resolution of ocular inflammation and decreased epitheliopathy as evidenced by improved homogeneity of light reflex on cornea.

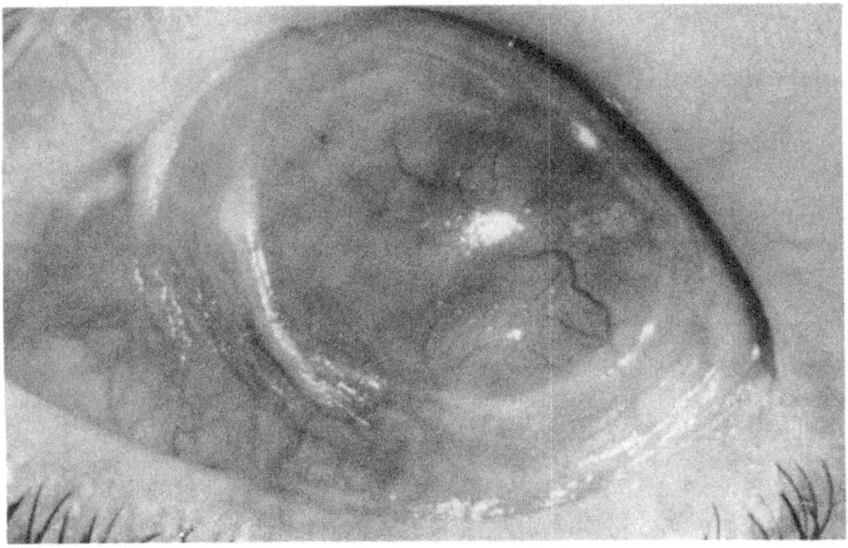

FIGURE 79: Same eye as in Fig 77, after systemic cyclosporine therapy. Ocular inflammation has abated, but patient is left with a scarred, vascularized cornea, and CF vision.

Current Status of Medical Therapy Program for CP

Our current approach to medical treatment of patients with active CP may be summarized as follows:

1. Sicca syndrome is treated aggressively. We favor ointment lubricants without preservatives (eg, Akwatears, Optilube, or Duolube ointments), applied at a frequency sufficient to maintain adequate surface lubrication and protection (eg, every 2 to 4 hours and at bedtime). Artificial tears without preservatives (eg, Refresh or Unisol drops) are employed as needed between ointment applications.

Topical retinoid (0.01% treitoin) ointment is used once or twice daily in one eye; we compare objective and subjective responses to the vitamin A ointment, and continue treatment beyond 4 weeks of therapy only if we and/or the patient conclude that there is a distinct therapeutic benefit to this agent. Fewer than 30% of our CP patients have shown an apparent benefit from typical retinoids. We strongly caution against inappropriate enthusiasm for the efficacy of this component of the therapeutic plan. We observed the unfortunate results of such inappropriate preoccupation with topical therapy for this systemic disease in three patients who are now functionally blind because the disease progressed while they were on topical retinoids.

2. Chronic blepharitis and meibomianitis are treated with vigorous lid hygiene and oral doxycycline, 100 mg once or twice daily. Manual expression of plugged meibomian ducts is performed at the time of every evaluation. Microbial colonizatin of the lids and meibomian glands by any organism, including Staphylococcus, is treated with appropriate topical and/or systemic antimicrobial agents. We have discovered two cases of chronic *Candida* infestation and one of Nocardia.

3. Chemotherapy for cases which are extremely active (4+)and rapidly progressive is begun with prednisone, 1 mg/kg, and cyclophosphamide, 2 mg/kg/day. The cyclophosphamide dose is adjusted according to therapeutic response, bone marrow response, and drug tolerance. Prednisone is gradually tapered, with a switch to alternate-day dosing by 8 to 12 weeks, and subsequent taper and discontinuation by 4 to 6 months. We presently maintain patients on chemotherapy for a minimum of 1 year.

Dapsone and prednisone are used for cases which are less active and which are not rapidly progressive. The initial daily dose of dapsone we employ is 2 mg/kg; the maximum dose ever employed is 200 mg/day. We emphasize that dapsone is not a benign drug. We follow our patients who are on dapsone as often and as carefully as we do those who are on cyclophosphamide. Patients who are not glucose-6-phosphate dehydrogenase-deficient as determined by the screening test, may still hemolyze when treated with dapsone, and therefore the hemoglobin, hematocrit, and reticulocyte count, as well as the white blood count, are important monitoring parameters for these patients. We usually accept a low degree of hemolysis if dapsone is achieving the desired therapeutic response. But reticulocytosis must adequately compensate for such hemolysis; a steadily falling hematocrit is unacceptable.

Approximately 70% of patients will respond well to dapsone. A large proportion of these (41% in our experience), will relapse within 6 months of cessation of dapsone therapy. We treat these patients with dapsone or with azathioprine. Azathioprine, 2 mg/kg initial dose, is also our second choice agent for the 30% of patients who do not respond adequately to dapsone. Adjustment of azathioprine dose is accomplished, as in the case of the other agents, through the judgment of the skilled chemotherapist, who, by virtue of training and experience is expert in the use of these agents.

CURRENT STATUS OF SURGICAL THERAPY FOR CP

Lids

Destruction of cilia follicles responsible for aberrant lash growth which produces damage to the ocular surface epithelium is crucial to the successful care of patients with CP not only because it eliminates one of the damaging elements, but also because it eliminates one variable that produces signs of conjunctival inflammation masking the extent of intrinsic, immunologically-driven inflammation, and hampering correct judgment regarding clinical response to chemotherapy. Mechanical epilation is inappropriate; lash regrowth is rapid, and the short, regrowing lash usually produces more damage to the ocular surface than did the original long lash. Electrolysis is acceptable, though it is tedious and the regrowth rate, in our experience, is approximately 30%.

Our routine therapy for trichiasis and distichiasis is cryoablation. Briefly, the eyelid is injected with 2% xylocaine with epinephrine (for vascular constriction and retardation of rewarming of the treated area). The nitrous oxide-cooled probe (KR Med Unit, Model MT 650, Cryomed, Inc, Bridgeport, CT) is applied to the lid margin for 40 seconds for each region to be treated. A repeat 40-second treatment application to each area is then followed by epilation. The recurrence rate, in our experience, is approximately 10%; we retreat areas of recurrence as described above.

Occlusion of inferior and superior canaliculi and lacrimal puncta is performed for any eye with Schirmer values (after topical anesthesia) of 2 mm or less on three successive occasions. Briefly, 2% xylocaine without epinephrine is injected into the lid around the punctum and canaliculus. A wire probe attached to an electric Hyphrecator is inserted into the canaliculus to its entry into the lacrimal sac. Application of the electrical current is begun and is continued until one observes contraction and blanching of the conjunctiva overlying the canaliculus. The probe is then withdrawn half-way and treatment is performed as described above. The probe is then removed from the canaliculus, the power is reduced to a setting of five, and the punctum is cauterized with the probe.

Ocular surgical procedures in general, and plastic surgical procedures in particular are notoriously unsuccessful in patients with active CP.[45] Such procedures, with rare exception, therefore should be deferred until successful control of disease activity has been achieved through systemic chemotherapeutic strategies. Quickert sutures or Weiss cautery procedures may provide temporary correction of entropion while systemic control of the disease is being achieved.

Once CP disease activity is controlled, marginal rotation of the eyelid, mucous membrane grafting, and fornix reconstruction (Figs 80 and 81) can be safely done, without significant danger of excessive postoperative inflammation and cicatrization.

Cornea

Corneal surgery almost always yields disappointing results in patients with CP. Most patients with CP keratopathy advanced enough to warrant keratoplasty also have irreversible mucosal keratinization and sicca syndrome sufficient to create an extremely poor prognosis for grafted corneal tissue. Rare exceptions to this exist, but keratoprosthesis is generally the only feasible alternative for corneal surgery and attempted visual rehabilitation. We have recently employed the Cardona keratoprosthesis, through the lid, in association with periosteal grafting (Fig 82a and b). This strategy has, to date, been modestly successful visually and has not been associated with the previously troublesome complications of prosthesis extrusion.

Lens

Most ophthalmologists have realized that cataract surgery performed on patients with ocular involvement of CP was usually followed by increased conjunctival inflammatory activity and rapid progression of conjunctival cicatrization and keratopathy. We have now performed extracapsular cataract extration with posterior chamber lens implantation in 23 patients with CP after successful abolition of all evidence of conjunctival inflammation through chemotherapy. The patients were maintained on chemotherapy for at least 6 months after surgery. Twenty-two of these patients have had successful cataract surgery and an uneventful recovery period, with restoration of vision to 20/50 or better as a result of the surgery. Only one of these patients has developed a problem postoperatively as a result of his pemphigoid. In this 64-year-old gentleman, who was on 150 mg of dapsone/day at the time of surgery, postoperative conjunctival inflammation escaped therapeutic control, and keratopathy with corneal ulcer development ensued before control could be reestablished with cyclophosphamide and prednisone. Corneal scarring and neovascularization resulted in a best corrected visual acuity of 20/300 in the operated eye.

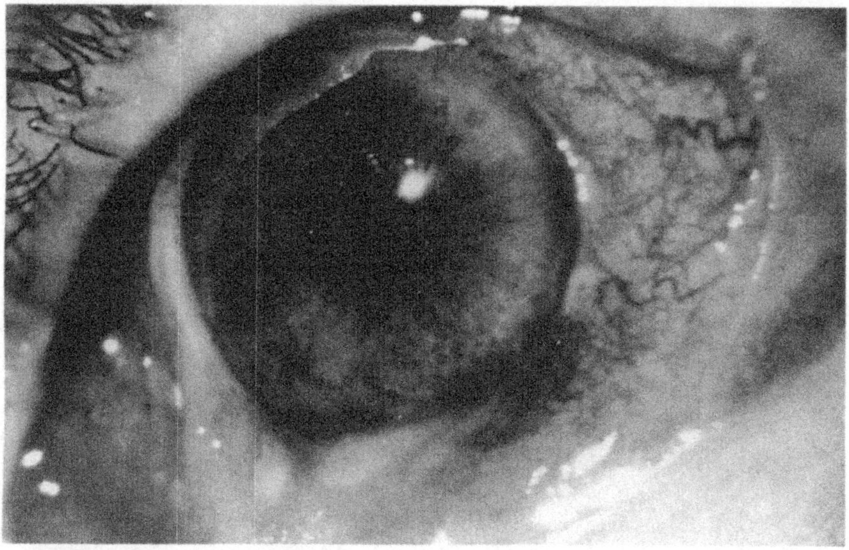

FIGURE 80: Stage III active CP, with nearly complete inferior fornix obliteration, and lagophthalmos with extensive inferior corneal exposure with keratopathy.

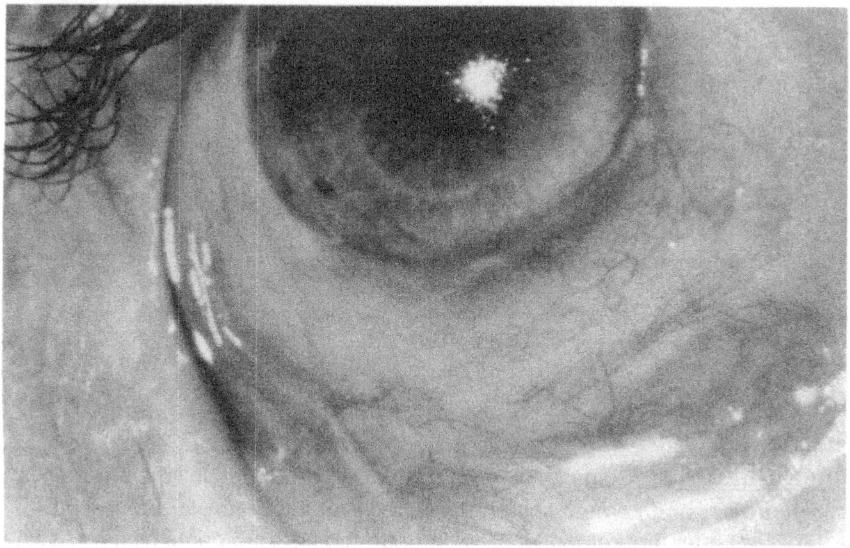

FIGURE 81: Same eye as in Fig 80, 6 months after institution of systemic cyclophosphamide therapy, and 2 months after inferior fornix reconstruction and mucosal membrane grafting. Lagophthalmos and inferior corneal exposure and keratopathy were corrected as a result of this surgery.

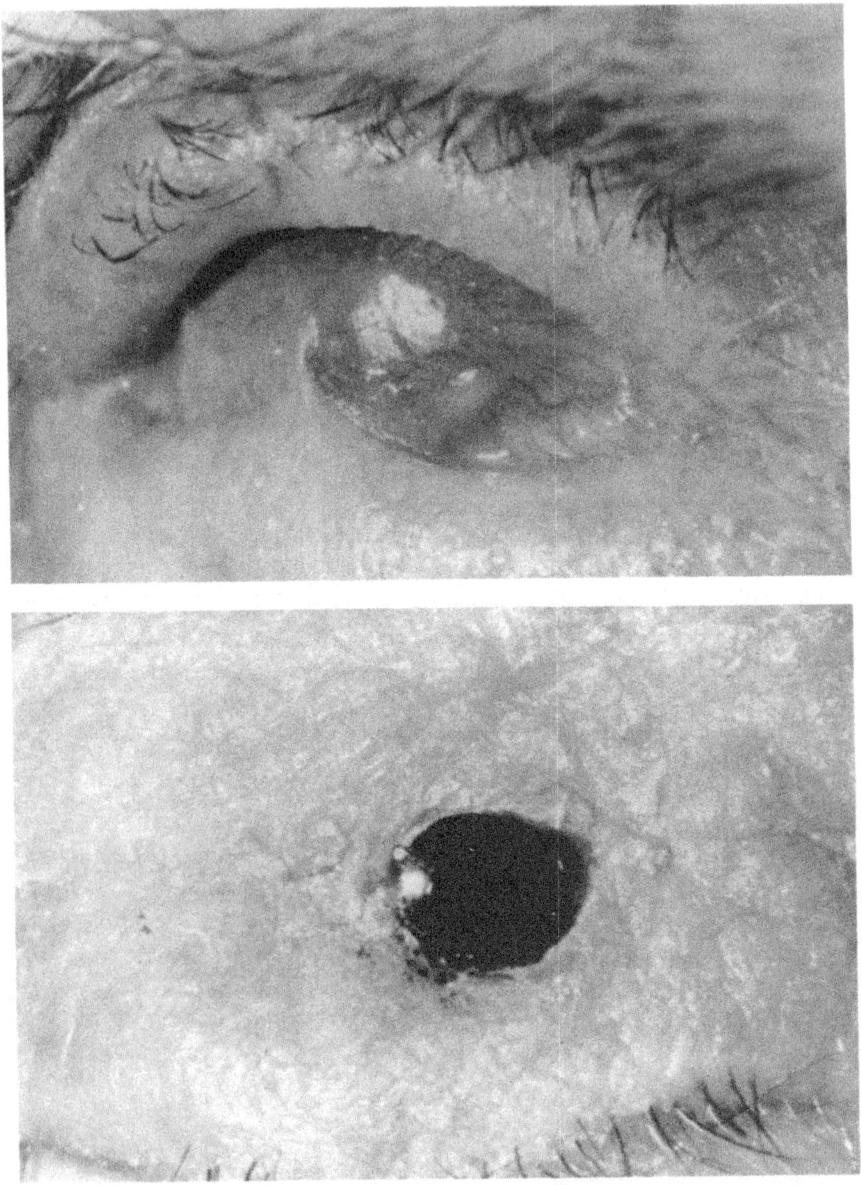

FIGURE 82: a: Stage IV CP with surface keratinization, extreme sicca syndrome, and corneal scarring and neovascularization. b: Same eye as in 82a, after performance of a through-the-lid keratoprosthesis. Visual rehabilitation from light perception to 20/100 has resulted in a substantial improvement in quality of this previously bilaterally blind patient's life.

Our perioperative management of CP patients includes oral prednisone, 1 mg/kg for 2 days prior to surgery and for 10 days postoperatively, in addition to maintaining the chemotherapeutic agent the patient is taking. Topical dexamethasone ointment, in addition to antibiotic ointment is also prescribed. The 10-0 nylon sutures, with buried knots, are not disturbed postoperatively unless unacceptable degrees of astigmatism are present, in which case a stitch which is cut is completely removed. No sutures are placed in the conjunctiva. Figs 83 through 86 show the right and left eyes of one of our CP patients, controlled for 10 months on cyclophosphamide prior to and following bilateral extracapsular cataract extraction and posterior chamber lens implantation; 5 months elapsed between the two operations.

SUMMARY, HYPOTHESIS, AND FUTURE DIRECTIONS

We studied 130 patients with biopsy-proven CP affecting the conjunctiva. Females outnumbered males, seven to four. The age range of the patients was 20 to 87 years. Forty-six percent of the patients had extraocular manifestations, and 12 of them had the potentially fatal complication of esophageal involvement. All of the patients had active, progressive disease, and 52 of the patients had suffered corneal complications of CP sufficient to impair vision to 20/200 or worse in at least one eye.

We confirmed the impression of others regarding an association with other autoimmune phenomena; 17.7% of our patients had another autoimmune disease, and 56 had circulating ANA. Our histopathologic studies disclosed two previously unreported notable features: mast cells are prominent participants in the conjunctival inflammatory reaction; and varying degrees of vasculopathy or frank vasculitis were frequently observed at the light and/or ultrastructural level. Our immunopathologic studies confirm the consistent feature of immunoreactant deposition at the epithelial BMZ, and show a derangement in the relative numbers of helper and suppressor T lymphocytes in the conjunctival substantia propria, suggesting the possibility of underregulation of inflammatory processes in the conjunctiva.

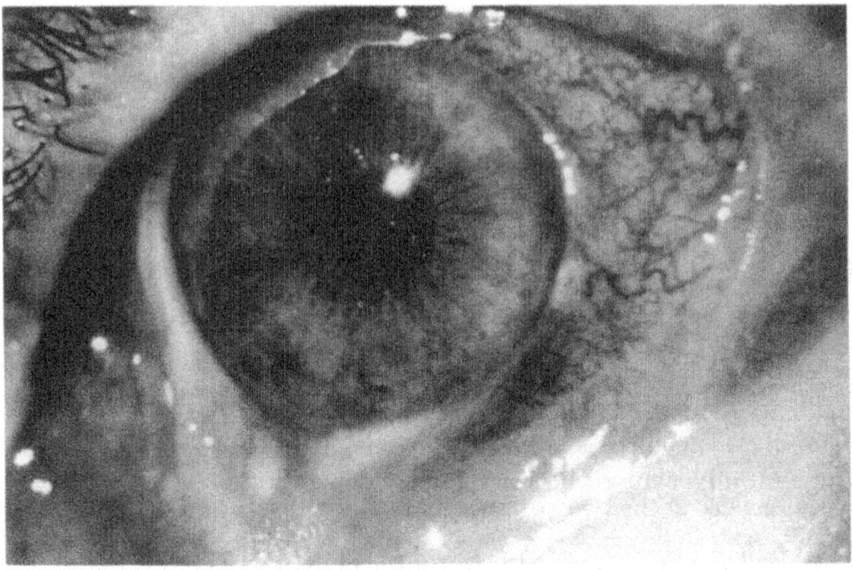

FIGURE 83: Right eye, stage III, active CP with peripheral corneal neovascularization nearly reaching pupillary margin inferiorly.

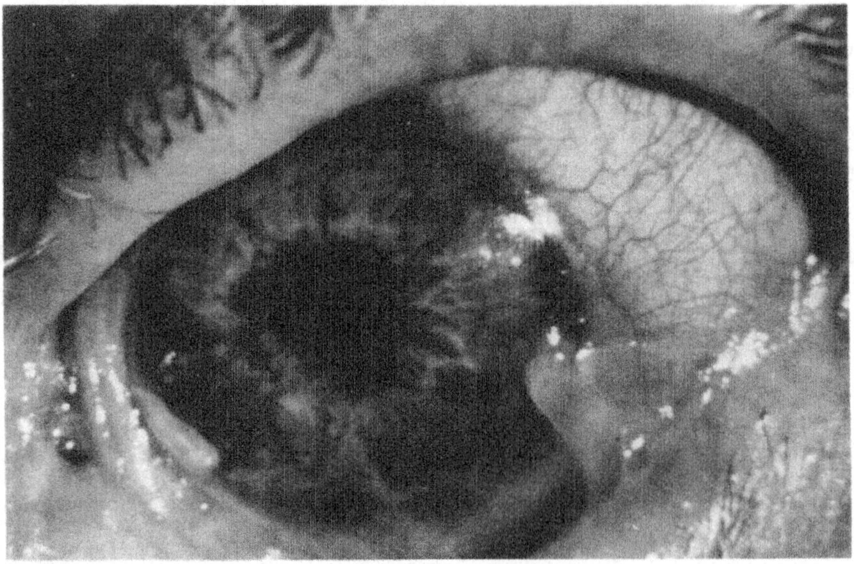

FIGURE 84: Same patient as in Fig 83, left eye, prior to institution of therapy

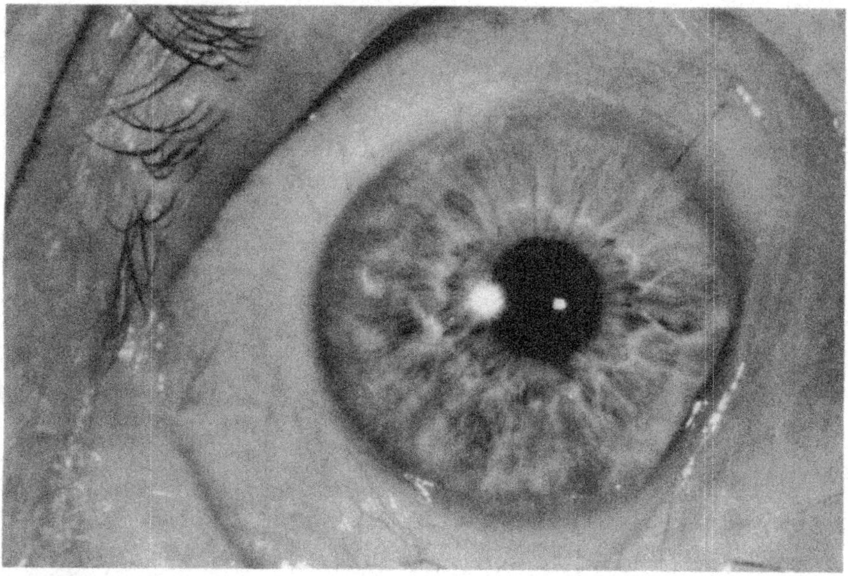

FIGURE 85: Right eye of patient in Fig 83, 8 weeks status after extracapsular cataract extraction and posterior chamber lens implantation while on chemotherapy for pemphigoid.

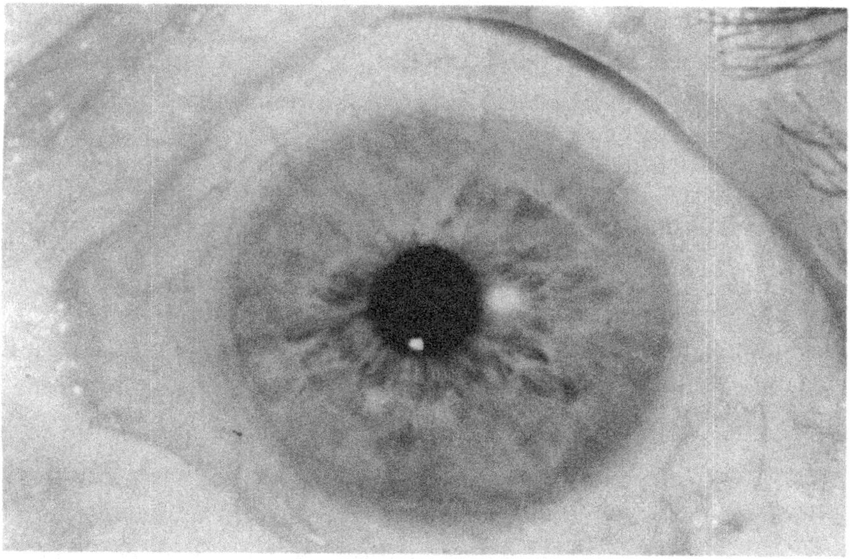

FIGURE 86: Left eye, same patient as in Fig 84, 10 weeks status after extracapsular cataract extraction and posterior chamber lens implantation while on maintenance chemotherapy.

We do not confirm the idea that tear and/or mucin deficiency is an important feature of CP, at least not until the disease is quite advanced. We found topical retinoids, lubricants, and steroids ineffective in controlling the inflammation and progressive cicatrization characteristic of progressive CP. Systemic prednisone controlled these latter features in 42% of patients treated with prednisone alone. Steroid-induced complications were substantial, however, and steroid taper was always associated with recurrence of disease activity.

Chemotherapy with dapsone, azathioprine, methotrexate or cyclophosphamide is highly effective in stopping CP disease activity. Cyclophosphamide is the most effective agent, in our experience, with 91% of our patients treated with this drug showing cessation of conjunctival inflammation and of progressive cicatrization. As of this writing, 58 patients treated with cyclophosphamide for at least 6 months have now been observed for at least 1 year after therapy has been stopped; 14 of these patients relapsed and required additional chemotherapy (usually with dapsone); 44 of the patients appeared cured.

Dapsone stopped all conjunctival inflammation and scarring in 70% of CP patients with mild-to-modest disease activity. Relapse after dapsone withdrawal was common, but the inflammation responded to reinstitution of dapsone or addition of azathioprine. The immunopathologic and histopathologic abnormalities characteristic of active CP were found to be reversible with successful systemic therapy if inflammation were abolished before extreme degrees of permanent structural alterations developed.

We hypothesize that a subtle defect in immunoregulation exists in this systemic autoimmune disease, with resultant production of autoantibody reactive with a component in the lamina lucida of the conjunctival epithelial BMZ. Antibody deposition at the BMZ, followed by activation of the complement pathway, results in a number of additional actions, including monocyte recruitment and activation and mast cell recruitment and degranulation (IgE-independent). The inflammatory mediators liberated from these cells recruit other cells, amplify the reaction, and induce bystander effects: vascular damage, fibroblast proliferation and collagen synthesis, and increased basal epithelial cell mitosis and squamous metaplasia. Corneal epitheliopathy develops secondary to inflammatory products in the tears and secondary to trichiasis and distichiasis which develops as a result of the subepithelial fibrosis. Meibomian gland dysfunction may result from inflammation and from scarring, and an alteration in the lipid component of the preocular tear film may play a role in TER, tear BUT, and corneal epitheliopathy. Progressive fibrosis results in lacrimal duct obstruction and increasing degrees of tear insufficiency in advanced cases. Mucin deficiency is also a late feature as the ocular surface epithelium becomes progressively keratinized.

Our work in this area continues in an effort to test this hypothesis and to develop more specific, yet effective therapy for CP. Our focus of attention has, until now, predominantly been on generalized immunosuppression to achieve effective suppression of inflammation and scarring and on use of agents like dapsone that affect peroxidase enzyme systems such as those present in monocytes, neutrophils, eosinophils, and mast cells. We, like others, suspected that the antibodies so characteristically present at the epithelial BMZ might simply represent an epiphenomenon, not a causal factor in CP. This concept has now changed.[112] Not only is the autoimmune status of CP now well established, but also it is now clear that the immune deposits are bound at sites where the earliest pathologic lesions are identified. Furthermore, two groups have now shown that circulating autoantibodies reactive with the lamina lucida of the BMZ can play a central role in lesion production.[113,114] Our further work will focus on techniques of immunomodulation designed to reestablish autotolerance without generalized immunosuppression.

REFERENCES

1. Foster CS: Immunosuppressive therapy in external ocular inflammatory disease. *Ophthalmology* 1980; 87:140-150.
2. Foster CS, Wilson LA, Ekins MB: Immunosuppressive therapy for progressive ocular cicatricial pemphigoid. *Ophthalmology* 1982; 89:340-353.
3. Lever WF: Pemphigus. *Medicine* 1953; 32:1-123.
4. Lever WF, Talbott JH: Pemphigus: A historical study. *Arch Dermatol Syph* 1942; 00:800-823.
5. Hippocrates: Hippocrates popularium liber sixtus, in JA vander Linden (ed): *Opera Omnia.* Apud Gaasbeekius, 1665, vol 1, p 798.
6. Koenig S: Lettre contenant plusieurs symptomes etrangers et surprenants, in F Planque (ed): *Bibliotheque Choisie de Medecine.* Paris, d'Houry, 1748-1770, vol 7, p 557
7. Wichmann JE: *Ideen zur Diagnostick.* Hannover, Helwing, 1793, vol 1, p 89
8. Cooper W: Pemphigus of the conjunctivae. *Ophthalmol Hosp Rep Lond Hosp Res* 1857; 1:155.
9. Thost A: Faile von Schleimhautpemphigus. *Deutsche Med Wochenschr* 1919; 45:477.
10. deSauvages FB: *Nosologia Methodica Sistens Morborum Classes.* Amsterdam, Fratres de Tournes, 1768, vol 1, p 430.
11. Duke-Elder S: *System of Ophthalmology.* St Louis, CB Mosby, 1965, vol 8, part 1, p 502.
12. von Graefe A: Ber *Dtsch Ophthalmol Ges* 1879; 12:234.
13. von Kries N: Caustistiche Mittheilungen aus der Augenklinik zu Halle: V. Essentialle Schrumpfung der Conjunctiva. *Arch Ophthalmol* 1878; 24:157-158.
14. Klauder JV, Cowan A: Ocular pemphigus and its relation to pemphigus of the skin and mucus membranes. *Am J Ophthalmol* 1942; 25:643-662.
15. Franke E: *Pemphigus und de essentialle Schrumpfung der Bindehart per des Auges.* Wiesbaden JF, Bergmann, 1900, p 111.
16. Bianco A: Cicatricial ocular pemphigus. *Am J Ophthalmo*l 1958; 46:881:884.
17. Rook A, Waddington E: Pemphigus and pemphigoid. *Br J Dermatol* 1953; 65:425-431.
18. Thost A: Chronic pemphigus of the mucus membranes. *Arch Laryn Rhin* 1911; 25:459-478.
19. Chaklkely TH: Chronic cicatricial conjunctivitis. *Am J Ophthalmol* 1969; 67:526-539.
20. Panebianco G, DiFede S: Mucous manifestations of otorhinolaryngologic in mucosynechiant and atrophic bullous dermatitis (so-called ocular pemphigus). *Boll Mal Orecch* 1964; 82:380-400.
21. Mondino BJ, Brown SI, Lempert S, et a!: The acute manifestations of ocular cicatricial pemphigoid: Diagnosis and treatment. *Ophthalmology* 1979; 86:543-555.
22. Mondino BJ, Brown SI: Ocular cicatricial pemphigoid. *Ophthalmology* 1981; 88: 95-100.

23. Bettelheim H. Kraft D, Zehetbauer G: Ober den sogenanneten Augenpemphigus (pemphigus ocularis; pemphigus conjunctivae). *Klin Auggenheilkd* 1972; 160:65-75.
24. Hardy WF, Lamb HD: Essential shrinking of the conjunctiva with report of two cases. *Am J Ophthalmol* 1917: 34:289-299.
25. Smith RC, Myers EA. Lamb HD: Ocular and oral pemphigus: Report of case with anatomic findings in eyeball. *Arch Ophthalmol* 1934; 11:635-640.
26. Bedell AJ: Ocular pemphigus: A clinical presentation. *Trans Am Ophthalmol Soc* 1964; 62:109-122.
27. Hardy KM, Perry HO, Pingree GC, et a!: Benign mucous membrane pemphigoid. *Arch Dermatol* 1911; 104:467-475.
28. Claussen W: T zur klinik des pemphigus conjunctivae. *Ber Zusammenkunft Dtsch Ophthalmol Ges* 1922; 43:251-256.
29. Eales H: Discussion of case report by Gunn RM: Case of pemphigus of conjunctiva in early stage. *Trans Ophthalmol Soc UK* 1892-93; 13:30-34.
30. Neeper ER: Conjunctival pemphigus: Improved following administration of Brook's hemoprotein. *Am J Ophthalmol* 1935; 18:363-364.
31. Foster CS: Ocular surface manifestations of neurologic and systemic disease. *Int Ophthalmol Clin* 1979; 19:207-242.
32. Pfluger E: Ueber pemphigus conjunctivae. *Klin Augenheilkd* 1878; 16:1-18.
33. Steffan XX: Pemphigus conjunctivae. *Klin Augenheilkd* 1885; 23:214-216.
34. Hanna R, Foster DR, Bean SF: Brunsting-Perry cicatricial pemphigoid associated with bullous pemphigoid. *J Am Acad Dermatol* 1980; 3:470-473.
35. Lever WF: *Pemphigus and Pemphigoid.* Springfield, IL, Charles C Thomas, 1965.
36. Shklar G, McCarthy PL: Oral lesions of mucous membrane pemphigus, a study of 85 cases. *Arch Otolaryngol* 1971; 93:354-364.
37. Person JR, Rogers RS III: Bullous and cicatricial pemphigoid: Clinical, histopathologic and immunopathologic correlations. *Mayo Clin Proc* 1977; 52:54-66.
38. Uhthoff W: Ueber einige bemerkenswerth Faile von Augenerkrankugen. *Klin Wochenschr* 1893; 30:251-252.
39. Anderson SR: Pemphigus of the conjunctiva with oral and cutaneous manifestations. *Acta Ophthalmol* (Kbh) 1958; 36:640-645.
40. Thost A: Ueber Schleimhautpemphigus. *Arch Laryngol Rhinol*1918; 31:599-631.
41. Custodis E: Die essentielle Bindehautschrumpfung des menschlichen. *Arch Ophthalmol* 1937; 137:364-418.
42. Tseng S, Hirst L, Maumenee A, et al: Possible mechanisms for the loss of goblet cells in mucin-deficient disorders. *Ophthalmology* 1984; 91:545-552.
43. Gazala JR: Ocular pemphigus. *Am J Ophthalmol* 1959; 48:355-362.
44. Anderson SR. Jensen OA, Kristensen EB, et al: Benign mucous membrane pemphigoid III: Biopsy. *Acta Ophthalmol* 1974; 52:455-463.

45. Mondino BJ: Bullous diseases of the skin and mucous membranes, in T Duane (ed): *Clinical Ophthalmology*. Philadelphia, Harper & Row, 1817, vol 4, chap 12.
46. Norn MS. Kristensen EB: Benign mucous membrane pemphigoid. II. Cytology. *Acta Ophthalmol* 1974; 52:282-290.
47. Carroll JM, Kuwahara T: Ocular pemphigus: An electron microscopic study of the conjunctival and corneal epithelium. *Arch Ophthalmol* 1968; 80:683-695.
48. Bean SF, Fusey N, West CE, et al: Ocular cicatricial pemphigoid (immunologic studies). *Trans Am Acad Ophthalmol Otolaryngol* 1976; 81:806-812.
49. Waltman SR. Yarian D: Circulating autoantibodies in ocular pemphigoid. *Am J Ophthalmol* 1974; 77:891-894.
50. Franklin RM, Fitzmorris CT: Antibodies against conjunctival basement membrane zone: Occurrence in cicatricial pemphigoid. *Arch Ophthalmol* 1983; 101:1611-1613.
51. Mondino BJ, Brown SI, Rabin BS: HLA antigens in ocular cicatricial pemphigoid. *Arch Ophthalmol* 1979; 97:479.
52. Furey N, West C, Andrews T, et al: Immunofluorescent studies of ocular cicatricial pemphigoid. *Am J Ophthalmol* 1975; 80:825-833.
53. Herron BE: Immunologic aspects of cicatricial pemphigoid. *Am J Ophthalmol* 1975; 79:271-278.
54. Mondino BJ, Ross AN, Rabin BS, et al: Autoimmune phenomena in ocular cicatricial pemphigoid. *Am J Ophthalmol* 1977; 83:443-450.
55. Mondino BJ, Brown SI, Rabin BS: Autoimmune phenomena of the external eye. *Ophthalmology* 1978; 85-801-817.
56. Kumar V, Yarborough C, Beutner EH: Complement-fixing intercellular antibodies in a case of cicatricial pemphigoid. *Arch Dermatol* 1980; 116:812-814.
57. Rogers RS III, Perry HO, Bean SF, et al: Immunopathology of cicatricial pemphigoid: Studies of complement deposition. *J Invest Dermatol* 1977; 68:39-43.
58. Laskaris G, Angelopoulos A: Cicatrial pemphigoid: Direct and indirect immunofluorescent studies. *Oral Surg* 1981; 51:48-54.
59. Spigel GT, Winkelmann RK: Cicatricial pemphigoid and rheumatoid arthritis. *Arch Dermatol* 1978; 114:415-417.
60. Redman RS, Thorne EG: Cicatricial pemphigoid in a patient with systemic lupus erythematosus. *Arch Dermatol* 1981; 117:109-110.
61. Krain LS, Bierman SM: Pemphigus vulgaris and internal malignancy. *Cancer* 1974; 33:1091-1099.
62. Skog E: Cutaneous manifestations associated with internal malignant tumors with particular reference to vesicular and bullous lesions. *Acta Dermatol Venereal* 1964; 44:114.
63. Curth HO: Cutaneous manifestations associated with malignant internal diseases, in *Dermatology in General Medicine*. 1st edition. New York, McGraw-Hill, 1971, pp 1561-1580.
64. Rook AJ: A pemphigoid eruption associated with carcinoma of the bronchus. *Trans St John's Hosp Dermatol Soc* 1968; 54:152-154.

65. Stone SP, Schroeter AL: Bullous pemphigoid and associated malignant neoplasms.*Arch Dermatol* 1975; 111:991-994.
66. Lim CC, MacDonald RH, Rook AJ: Dermatitis herpetiformis and pemphigoid eruptions in the elderly. *Trans St John's Hosp Dermatol Soc* 1968; 54:148-151.
67. Greer KE, Beacham BE, Askew FC: Benign mucous membrane pemphigoid in association with internal malignancy. *Cutis* 1980; 25:183-185.
68. Lever WF, Schaumburg-Lever G: Immunosuppressants and prednisone in pemphigus vulgaris: Therapeutic results obtained in 63 patients between 1961 and 1975. *Arch Dermatol* 1977; 113:1236-1241.
69. Wolff K: Immunosuppressive therapy. *Bull Dermatosen Hautarzt* (Suppl) 1976; 1:25.
70. Fellner MJ, Katz JM, McCabe JB: Successful use of cyclophosphamide and prednisone for initial treatment of pemphigus vulgaris. *Arch Dermatol* 1978; 114:889-894.
71. Dave VK, Vickers CFH: Azathioprine in the treatment of mucocutaneous pemphigoid. *Br J Dermatol* 1974; 90:183-186.
72. Brody HJ, Pirozzi DJ: Benign mucous membrane pemphigoid: Response to therapy with cyclophosphamide. *Arch Dermatol* 1977; 113:1598-1599.
73. Rook A, Waddington E: Pemphigus and pemphigoid. *Br J Dermatol*1953; 65:425-431.
74. Person JR, Rogers RS III: Bullous pemphigoid responding to sulfapyridine and the sulfones. *Arch Dermatol* 1977; 113:610-615.
75. Rogers RS III, Seehafer JR, Perry HO: Treatment of cicatricial (benign mucous membrane) pemphigoid with dapsone. *J Am Acad Dermatol* 1982; 6:215-223.
76. Dohlman CH, Lemp MA, English FP: Dry eye syndromes. *Int Ophthalmol Clin* 1970; 10:215-251.
77. Lamberts DW, Foster CS, Perry HD: Schirmer test after topical anesthesia and the tear meniscus height in normal eyes. *Arch Ophthalmol* 1979; 97:1082-1085.
78. Lemp MA, Hamill J: Factors affecting tear film breakup in normals. *Arch Ophthalmol* 1973; 89:103-105.
79. Lemp MA: Breakup of the tear film. *Int Ophthalmol Clin* 1973; 13:97-102.
80. —The mucin-deficient dry eye. *Int Ophthalmol Clin* 1973; 13:185-189.
81. Thoft RA, Friend J, Kinoshita MA, et a!: Ocular cicatricial pemphigoid associated with hyperproliferation of the conjunctival epithelium. *Am J Ophthalmol* 1984; 98:37-42.
82. Charles A, Smiddy GF: Fibrils of the human epidermis. *J Invest Dermatol* 1957; 29:327-338.
83. Morjan LC, Pratley JN: Differential effects of tripsin on the epidermis of Rana catesbeiana: Observations on differentiating junctions and cytoskeletons. *Cell Tissue Res* 1979; 198:349-362.

84. Cavanagh HD, Colley AM: Cholinergic, adrenergic, and PGE sub-1 effects on cyclic nucleotides and growth in cultured corneal epithelium. *Metab Pediatr Syst Ophthalmol* 1982; 6:63-74.
85. Patten JT, Cavanagh HD, Allansmith MR: Induced ocular pseudopemphigoid. *Am J Ophthalmol* 1976; 82:272-276.
86. Hirst LW, Werblin T, Novak M: Drug induced cicatrizing conjunctivitis simulating ocular pemphigoid. *Cornea* 1982; 1:121-128.
87. Lass JH, Thoft RA, Dahlman CH: Idoxyuridine-induced conjunctival cicatrization. *Arch Ophthalmol* 1983; 101:747-750.
88. Norn MS: Pemphigoid related to epinephrine treatment. *Am J Ophthalmol* 1977;83:138.
89. Rahi AH, Chapman CM, Garner A, et al: Pathology of practolol induced ocular toxicity. *Br J Ophthalmol* 1976; 60:312-323.
90. Wintroub BU, Mihm MC, Goetzel EJ, et al: Morphologic and functional evidence for release of mast cell products in bullous pemphigoid. *J Engl J Med* 1978; 298:417-421.
91. Dvorak AM, Mihm MC, Oshee JE, et al: Bullous pemphigoid, an ultrastructural study of the inflammatory response: Eosinophil, basophil, and mast cell granular changes in multiple biopsies from one patient. *J Invest Dermatol* 1982; 78:91-101.
92. Carter RD, Joyner WL, Renkin EM: Effects of histamine and some other substances in molecular activity of the capillary wall to plasma proteins in dextran. *Microb Res* 1974; 7:31-48.
93. Susi FR, Shklar G: Histochemistry and fine structure of oral lesions of mucous membrane pemphigoid. *Arch Dermatol* 1911; 104:224-253.
94. Greiner JV, Korb DR, Covington HI, et al: Human ocular mucus, scanning electron microscopic study. *Arch Ophthalmol* 1982; 100:1614-1617.
95. Pfiter RR: The normal surface of corneal epithelium: A scanning electron microscopic study. *Invest Ophthalmol* 1973; 12:654-668.
96. Hazlett LD, Wells P, Spann B, et al: Epithelial desquamation in the adult mouse cornea: A correlative scanning and transmission microscopy study. *Ophthalmic Res* 1980; 12:315-323.
97. Mollenhauer HH: Plastic embedding mixtures for use in electron microscopy. *Stain Technol* 1964; 39:111-114.
98. Greiner JV, Covington HI, Allansmith MR: The human limbus, a scanning electron microscopic study. Arch *Ophthalmol* 1979; 97:1159-1165.
99. Greiner JV, Covington HI, Allansmith MR: Surface morphology of giant papillary conjunctivitis in contact lens wearers. *Am J Ophthalmol* 1978; 85:242-252.
100. Marriott C, Beeson MF, Brown DT: Biopolymer induced changes in mucus viscoelasticity, in EN Chantler, JB Elder, M Elstein (eds): *Mucus in Health and Disease*. Part II. New York, Plenum Press, 1900, pp 89-92.
101. Ralph RA: Conjunctival goblet cell density in normal subjects and in dry eye syndromes. *Invest Ophthalmol* 1975; 14:299-302.

102. Kinoshita S, Kiorpes TC, Friend J, et al: Goblet cell density in ocular surface disease, a better indicator than tear mucin. *Arch Ophthalmol* 1983; 101:1284-1287
103. Nelson JD, Wright JC: Conjunctival goblet cell densities in ocular surface disease. *Arch Ophthalmol* 1984; 102:1049-1051.
104. Dohlman CH, Friend J, Kalerar V, et al: The glycoprotein (mucus) content of tears from normal and dry eye patients. *Exp Eye Res* 1976; 22:359-365.
105. Gillette TE, Allansmith MR, Greiner JV, et al: Histologic and immunohistologic comparison of main and accessory lacrimal gland tissue. *Am J Ophthalmol* 1980; 89:724-730.
106. Greiner JV, Kenyon KR, Henriquez AS, et al: Mucus secretory vesicles in the conjunctival epithelium of wearers of contact lenses. *Arch Ophthalmol* 1980; 98: 1843-1846.
107 Greiner JV, Weidman TA, Korb DR, et al: Histochemical analysis of secretory vesicles in nongoblet conjunctival epithelial cells. *Acta Ophthalmol* 1985; 63:89-92.
108. Dilly PN, Mackie IA: Surface changes in the anesthetic conjunctiva in man, with special reference to the production of mucus from a nongoblet-cell source. *Br J Ophthalmol* 1981; 65:833-842.
109. Kawano K, Uehara F, Sameshima M, et al: Application of lectins for detection of goblet cell carbohydrates of the human conjunctiva. *Exp Eye Res* 1984; 38:439-447.
110. Chao CW, Vergnes JP, Brown SI: Fractionation and partial characterization of macromolecular components from human ocular mucus. *Exp Eye Res* 1983; 36:139-150
111. Moore JC, Tiffany JM: Human ocular mucus: Origins and preliminary characterization. *Exp Eye Res* 1979; 29:291-301.
112. Katz SI: Blistering skin diseases. *N Engl J Med* 1985; 313:1657-1658.
113 Anhalt GJ, Bahn CF, Labib RS, et a!: Pathogenic effects of bullous pemphigoid autoantibodies on rabbit corneal epithelium. *J Clin Invest* 1981; 68:1097-1101.
114. Gammon WR, Merritt CC, Lewis DM, et a!: An in vitro model of immune complex- mediated basement membrane zone separation caused by pemphigoid antibodies, leukocytes, and complement. *J Invest Dermatol* 1982; 78:285-290

APPENDIX I

CP INTAKE PROTOCOL—GENERAL

History
Eye examination
Photography
Laboratory—complete blood count; sedimentation rate
Urinalysis
Autoantibody screen and immune complexes
HLA typing
Glucose-6-phosphate dehydrogenase screen
Tear & mucus collection
Selected patients—TER
Impression cytology
Tear production
Tear osmolarity
Biopsy
Education—instruction
—Educational material
Return visit -Questions answered
-Review of data
-Treatment plan

APPENDIX II

CP HISTORY AND EXAMINATION DATA FORM

Name:	Date of birth:
Address:	SS #:
Telephone:	Insurance:
Examination date:	Referred by:

Ocular history
Summary of ocular drug use
Summary of ocular surgery

Medical history
Skin lesions
Mucous membranes
- Nose
- Mouth
- Pharynx
- Larynx
- Esophagus
- Vagina
- Urethra
- Anus

Medicines
Allergies
Ocular examination
External examination
- Lids—Skin
  - Entropion
  - Lagophthalmos
- Lashes—Trichiasis
  - Distichiasis
- EOM's & Bell's phenomenon
- Pupils
- Conjunctival injection

Slit lamp examination
- Lid margins
- Meibomian ducts
- Punctae
- Conjunctiva—
  - Cells and fluid
  - Fibrosis
  - Fornix foreshortening
  - Symblepharon formation
  - Ankyloblepharon
  - Rose-Bengal stain
  - Fluorescein stain
- Cornea—
  - Epitheliopathy
  - Stroma
  - Endothelium
  - Neovascularization
  - Sensation
- Anterior chamber
- Iris
- Lens
- Vitreous
- Fundus (dilated)

APPENDIX III
CP DIAGNOSTIC LABORATORY DATA FORM

Date:
Biopsy: IF
ABC
JB-4
Date:
Schirmer, with anesthetic:
Tear osmolarity:
Tear evaporation:
Impression cytology:
Urinary sediment:

WBC/Hct:
Segs:
Lymphs:
Monos:
Eos:
Baso:
Platelet:

ANA	αBMZ	αMitochondrial	αSmooth muscle
RF	Raji cell	C1q binding	
HLA			

APPENDIX IV
HISTOPATHOLOGY DATA FORM

Patient name:
Biopsy date:
Eye:

Epithelium— Cell layers
Squamous metaplasia
Balloon degeneration
Goblet cells: Field 1 ____ Field 2 ____ Field 3 ____

Inflammatory cells Field 1 ____ Field 2 ____ Field 3 ____
Plasma cell
Lymphocyte
Histiocyte
Mast cell
Mast cell degran.
Eosinophil
Neutrophil
Other

Vasculitis

Perivasculitis

Comments

APPENDIX V
THERAPY MONITORING DATA FORM

Date:

Symptoms
- Fatigue
- Malaise
- Dysphagia
- Anorexia
- Nausea
- Vomiting
- Dyspnea
- Dysuria

- Other

Urine sediment
Hemogram
WBC
- Segs
- Lymphs
- Monos
- Eos
- Baso
- Platelet

HgB
Hct
- BUN
- Creatinine
- SGOT
- SGPT
- LDH
- Alkaline phosphatase

ABOUT THE AUTHOR

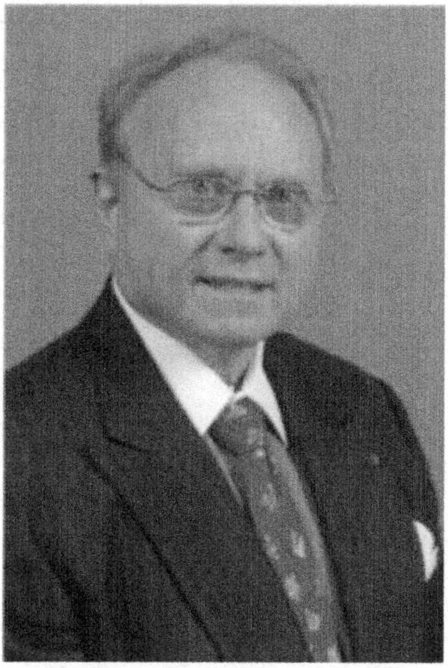

Dr. Foster was born and raised in West Virginia, received his Bachelor of Science Degree in Chemistry at Duke University, with Distinction and Phi Beta Kappa in 1965, and received his Doctor of Medicine at Duke University Medical Center, in 1969, being elected to Alpha Omega Alpha. He trained in Internal Medicine at Duke University Hospital from 1969-1970, and at the National Heart and Lung Institute, at the Nation Institutes of Health in Bethesda, Maryland, from 1970 to 1972, during which time he also taught Internal Medicine, with an appointment as Instructor in Medicine at the George Washington University Hospital in Washington, DC.

In 1972, Dr. Foster entered his Ophthalmology Residency training program at Washington University (Barnes Hospital), in St. Louis, Missouri, and having completed that in 1975, traveled to Boston to do two additional Fellowship trainings in Cornea and External Diseases, and in Ocular Immunology. He completed this training in 1977 and was invited to join the full-time faculty of the Department of Ophthalmology of Harvard Medical School, where he was a member of the Cornea Service and Director of Residency Training Program at the Massachusetts Eye and Ear Infirmary. He began his independent research in 1977 and has since been continuously funded by grants from the National Institutes of Health.

After 30 years on the full time faculty of Massachusetts Eye and Ear Infirmary, in 2005 he decided to establish his own private practice—The Massachusetts Eye Research and Surgery Institution, a state of the art practice dedicated to eye inflammatory diseases with its own chemotherapy infusion suite, blood, and pathology laboratories. Dr. Foster continues to direct a research laboratory at the Massachusetts Eye Research and Surgery Institution (MERSI), through the support of his research foundation, The Ocular Immunology and Uveitis Foundation, and continues his teachings activities and training fellows as a Clinical Professor of Ophthalmology (PT) at Harvard Medical School. He has also authored over 1,000 published medical papers and 8 textbooks.

Made in the USA
Monee, IL
04 November 2026

67377028R00095